'Positive health is a new paradigm, a shift in healthcare from just the diagnosis of disease and treatment of illness to include sustainable selfcare strategies through the science of flourishing. The authors provide a much needed holistic focus on what's strong as opposed to what's wrong, on how health and wellbeing can be developed and supported. Leveraging the emerging evidence from lifestyle medicine and positive psychology this book provides the why as well as the how in terms of positive change. If you are involved in healthcare, education, training or simply are curious to learn how to add more life to your years, then this book is for YOU!'

**Mark Rowe**, *PhD, author of The Vitality Mark*

'Positive health: The Basics provides excellent insights to the way we all should approach health and wellbeing. Promoting the positive can negate the negative and so positive health is for everyone, regardless of how high or low we are on the wellbeing continuum.'

**Darren Morton**, *PhD, director of the Lifestyle Medicine and Health Research Centre, Avondale University, creator of The Lift Project*

'The authors are modest when they describe this work as "The Basics". It is much more than that. Health professionals and others who want to understand more about thriving in life will find a foundation for understanding and action in positive health. The disciplines of lifestyle medicine, salutogenesis and positive psychology are deftly woven into the philosophical framework of not simply "health", but what it means to live life well.'

**Simon Matthews**, *FACLM, MHlthSc, DipIBLM, NBC-HWC*

'All of us can benefit from the "positive health: The Basics" in order to leverage our full potential – not only to prevent and treat mental and physical conditions, but also become our best selves, regardless of the adversities we may face. individually and supporting an environment for a health-sustaining and positive future globally. I commend the authors for pulling together the key basics of positive health and making it accessible in this text.'

**Liana Lianov**, *MD, MPH, president of Global Positive Health Institute, author of* Strengths in the Mirror, co-author of Lifestyle Medicine From the Inside Out

'First, this is a great book, easy to read and important. Well done. The authors take the reader through the concepts and theories of positive psychology and the pillars of ACLM learn about positive health. The reader is provided tangible tools to wellbeing. Medicine will change.'

**Kathi Norman**, *PhD, creator of Positive Medicine*

# POSITIVE HEALTH

This introductory book offers a clear guide to the new field of Positive Health, which incorporates a shift towards perceiving body and mind as an integrated system. The book combines lifestyle medicine research and practice, such as healthy eating, good sleep hygiene, and physical activity, with positive psychology research and practice, including cognitive, arts-based, and positive affect tools, to delve into the psychology of positive health, physiology, and health behaviour.

Combining theory with interventions, and illustrated by case material, mind-maps, and infographics, the book also provides exercises on how to use key research findings from the field of positive health to enhance personal wellbeing. It helps readers focus on the changes they can make to their thinking, attitudes, and behaviours, as well as changes they can instigate in their environment that can lead to positive health. Topics covered include the social determinants of health and meaning as a factor contributing to health.

It is essential for introductory courses on positive health, and supplementary reading for courses on positive psychology or wellbeing, as well as valuable reading for all healthcare professionals and policy makers.

**Dr Jolanta Burke** is a chartered psychologist (BPS), an award-winning researcher specialising in positive psychology and a senior lecturer (US: associate professor) at the Centre for positive health Sciences. She leads a Good Life research lab, and her team explores ways in which positive activities can be applied to maximise health and wellbeing impact. She was acknowledged by the Irish Times as one of 30 people who make Ireland a better place. For more information, go to: www.jolantaburke.com.

**Dr Pádraic J. Dunne** is an immunologist (research scientist), a practising psychotherapist, an accredited senior coach, and a certified lifestyle medicine professional, based at the RCSI Centre for Positive Health Sciences (CPHS). As a senior lecturer (US: associate professor) and lead researcher of the Digital Health Research Group, he is interested in the development of health coach-led health and wellbeing programmes for the general public, healthcare workers, and citizens with a chronic disease diagnosis.

**Dr Elaine Byrne** has held academic positions at the University of Pretoria in South Africa, the RCSI University of Medicine and Health Sciences in Ireland, and the University of Oslo in Norway. Her research interests revolve around supporting healthy people in healthy societies and organisations, with a focus on areas such as addressing self-stigma around HIV, global health systems and health services research, and qualitative research methodology.

**Professor Ciaran A. O'Boyle** is Director of the centre and a professor of psychology at the RCSI University of Medicine and Health Sciences with over 35 years' experience as an educator, researcher, and trainer. He established the RCSI Department of Psychology in 1985, the RCSI Institute of Leadership in 2005, and the RCSI Centre for Positive Psychology and Health in 2019.

# The Basics Series

The Basics is a highly successful series of accessible guidebooks which provide an overview of the fundamental principles of a subject area in a jargon-free and undaunting format.

Intended for students approaching a subject for the first time, the books both introduce the essentials of a subject and provide an ideal springboard for further study. With over 50 titles spanning subjects from artificial intelligence (AI) to women's studies, The Basics are an ideal starting point for students seeking to understand a subject area.

Each text comes with recommendations for further study and gradually introduces the complexities and nuances within a subject.

**EVOLUTIONARY PSYCHOLOGY**
Will Reader and Lance Workman

**WORK PSYCHOLOGY**
Laura Dean and Fran Cousans

**Forensic Psychology (3rd Edition)**
Sandie Taylor

**APHASIA**
Jane Marshall

**POSITIVE HEALTH**
Jolanta Burke, Pádraic J. Dunne, Elaine Byrne, and
Ciaran A. O'Boyle

For more information about this series, please visit: www.routledge.com/Routledge-The-Basics-Series/book-series/B

# POSITIVE HEALTH

# THE BASICS

Jolanta Burke, Pádraic J. Dunne,
Elaine Byrne, and Ciaran A. O'Boyle

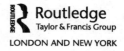

LONDON AND NEW YORK

Designed cover image: Getty Images via Slanapotam

First published 2025
by Routledge
4 Park Square, Milton Park, Abingdon, Oxon OX14 4RN

and by Routledge
605 Third Avenue, New York, NY 10158

*Routledge is an imprint of the Taylor & Francis Group, an informa business*

*British Library Cataloguing-in-Publication Data*
A catalogue record for this book is available from the British Library

*Library of Congress Cataloging-in-Publication Data*
Names: Burke, Jolanta, author. | Dunne, Pádraic J., author. | Byrne,
Elaine, author. | O'Boyle, Ciaran A., author.
Title: Positive health : the basics / Jolanta Burke, Padraic J. Dunne,
Elaine Byrne, and Ciaran A. O'Boyle.
Description: Abingdon, Oxon ; New York, NY : Routledge, 2025. |
Series: The basics | Includes bibliographical references and index.
Identifiers: LCCN 2024034295 (print) | LCCN 2024034296 (ebook) |
ISBN 9781032600123 (hardback) | ISBN 9781032600116 (paperback) |
ISBN 9781003457169 (ebook)
Subjects: LCSH: Positive psychology. | Well-being.
Classification: LCC BF204.6 .B865 2025 (print) | LCC BF204.6 (ebook) |
DDC 150.19/88—dc23/eng/20240813
LC record available at https://lccn.loc.gov/2024034295
LC ebook record available at https://lccn.loc.gov/2024034296

ISBN: 978-1-032-60012-3 (hbk)
ISBN: 978-1-032-60011-6 (pbk)
ISBN: 978-1-003-45716-9 (ebk)

DOI: 10.4324/9781003457169

Typeset in Bembo
by SPi Technologies India Pvt Ltd (Straive)

To our readers, may this book help you live a contented and healthy life.

# CONTENTS

# FOREWORD

## ADVANCING POSITIVE HEALTH WITH THE BASICS

In our rapidly changing and increasingly challenging society, every individual, organisation, and community has the potential to thrive by adapting and integrating key elements of positive health. This book provides a grounding for understanding the emerging and evolving field of positive health based in the science of lifestyle medicine and positive psychology. The basic theories and practical interventions are explained in a user-friendly way, highlighted with relatable case examples. Leaders of organisations, professionals, and individuals can apply these lessons in various contexts to promote positive health for their employees, members, families, and themselves.

Whilst more research is needed to uncover best practices in positive health for different populations, cultures, and contexts, the richness of current available tools and approaches reviewed here offers an opportunity to begin to harness their power immediately. Chapters spotlight how the positive health approach can improve physical health, mental health, and total wellbeing. In addition to delineating more well-known approaches, such as mind–body practices, this book uncovers exciting new areas of research and practice, such as the role of the microbiome and epigenetics. Moreover, the role of the six lifestyle medicine pillars and ways to harness positive psychology and positive health in healthy behaviours and coaching are explored.

All of us can benefit from the positive health basics in order to leverage our full potential – not only to prevent and treat mental and physical conditions, but also to become our best selves, regardless of the adversities we may face. As an advocate for transforming health and healthcare by working along two continua – one that moves us from disease to health (illness continuum) and another that moves us from loneliness, stress, and trauma towards becoming our best selves (positive health continuum), I'm a keen fan of the principles highlighted here. These principles can be used by individuals, organisations, and across communities for boosting our wellbeing individually and supporting an environment for a health-sustaining and positive future globally.

I commend the authors for pulling together the key basics of positive health and making it accessible in this text. By collectively applying these basics, I am optimistic we can all travel on the life-long journey of positive health.

Liana Lianov, MD, MPH
President, Global Positive Health Institute
Author, *Strengths in the Mirror*
Co-author, *Lifestyle Medicine From the Inside Out*

# ABOUT THE RCSI CENTRE

The Royal College of Surgeons in Ireland (RCSI), University of Medicine and Health Sciences is committed to advancing education, fostering growth, and making significant discoveries to improve human health. As a leading international institution in health sciences education and research, RCSI offers a range of undergraduate and postgraduate programmes across various health sciences disciplines. With a global footprint that includes campuses in Bahrain, Dubai, and Malaysia and its main campus in Dublin, RCSI hosts a diverse student body from over 60 countries. Studying at RCSI not only provides a comprehensive education but also offers unique opportunities for global networking and exposure to diverse healthcare systems.

RCSI's commitment to excellence is reflected in its rankings. We are proud to be in the top 2% of the Times Higher Education World University Rankings, a testament to the quality of our education and research. Furthermore, we hold the 1st position worldwide for social and economic impact under the United Nations' Sustainable Development Goal (SDG) 3 'Good Health and Well-being' (2023 Times Higher Education World University Rankings), highlighting our dedication to making a positive difference in the world.

The RCSI Centre for positive health Sciences (CPHS), established in 2019, specialises in health and wellbeing. Our mission is to educate, nurture, and discover ways to improve health and wellbeing through positive psychology and lifestyle medicine. CPHS is a centre of innovation, providing evidence-based resources to deepen the understanding of how behaviour influences health outcomes, and empowering individuals and communities to take control of their health.

We offer various educational programmes, including the Postgraduate Diploma in Positive Health, Master's in Positive Health Coaching, Professional Diploma in Leading Workplace Health and Well-being, Master's in Applied Positive Psychology (Health), and Micro-credential certificate offering an Introduction to lifestyle medicine. Additionally, we provide free Science of Health and Happiness programmes for adults, seniors, and young people. We have also recently established a free online positive health-based initiative (The Motherhood Programme) which offers practical educational support to people who are pregnant, new parents, and their families and friends.

We conduct unique research at our centre in three distinct areas:

1. Positive health coaching and digital health platforms
2. Pathways to living a good life
3. Arts and positive mental health

The following are the recent books published by the RCSI Centre for Positive Health Sciences about positive health:

1. Burke, J., Dunne, P.J., Meehan, T., O'Boyle, C. A., & Nieuwerburgh, C. (2023). *Positive health: 100+ research-based positive psychology and lifestyle medicine tools for improving wellbeing.* Routledge.
2. Burke, J., Boniwell, I., Frates, B., Lianov, L., & O'Boyle, C. A. (2024). *International Routledge handbook for positive health sciences: Positive psychology and lifestyle medicine research and practice.* Routledge.
3. Lianov, L., & Burke, J. (2024). *Lifestyle medicine from the inside out: Using positive psychology and healthy lifestyles for positive health.* Routledge.
4. Burke, J., Dunne, P.J., Byrne, J., & O'Boyle, C. A. (2024). *Positive health: The basics.* Routledge.
5. Burke, J. & Lianov, L. (in preparation). *Positive health from A to Z.* Routledge.

For more information about the centre, go to: https://www.rcsi.com/cphs

# INTRODUCTION TO POSITIVE HEALTH

*Emily prided herself on her physical health. She ran daily, ate well, and rarely fell ill. To her, health meant not being sick.*

*However, Emily began feeling stressed at work, struggling to sleep, and constantly on edge. She dismissed these feelings, believing she was healthy as long as she was not physically ill.*

*One evening, her friend Sarah asked, "How are you doing, Emily?"*

*"I am healthy. I am not sick", Emily replied.*

*"But are you well? You seem stressed and unhappy", Sarah responded.*

*This puzzled Emily. She had never considered health beyond the absence of illness. Sarah explained that proper health includes mental and emotional wellbeing, defined by the World Health Organisation (WHO) as "complete physical, mental, and social wellbeing, not merely the absence of disease."*

*Curious, Emily realised she had been neglecting her mental health. She started practising mindfulness, talking to a therapist, and pursuing hobbies. Gradually, her mood and overall wellbeing improved.*

*Emily's story shows the limitations of viewing health only as the absence of illness. By adopting a holistic approach, she found a more balanced and fulfilling life, embracing the broader concept of health advocated by the WHO. This shift enabled her to lead a more vibrant and meaningful life, embodying wellbeing.*

Most of us tend to think about our health in terms of two opposing categories: "health" and "illness". We consider ourselves healthy if we are not suffering from an illness or disease. From a Western perspective, this way of thinking has a long tradition and is the basis for most health professionals' understanding of illness and their

DOI: 10.4324/9781003457169-1

approach to healthcare (Engel, 1977; Leonardi, 2018). Additionally, especially in the West, we often see mental and physical functioning as separate and distinct, making a distinction between "mental" health and "physical" health (Lai & Chang, 2022). This binary paradigm shapes our understanding of health and influences our health behaviours. For instance, it may lead us to neglect our mental health if we are physically well, or vice versa. There is need for a more holistic view of health that encompasses all aspects of wellbeing, which is what positive health can offer.

This Western binary paradigm of health and illness, while deeply ingrained, has its limitations. It is reflected in most formal healthcare systems, which have evolved primarily to treat illness and disease once they occur, with much less focus on prevention or optimising health and wellbeing. The goals of most healthcare systems within this binary paradigm are to cure or rehabilitate the patient, prevent further deterioration, and optimise quality of life, especially for those with chronic or progressive conditions. While these approaches are vital in the context of disease and illness, they offer limited value for those who are not suffering from an illness or disease but are not exactly thriving either.

Despite this approach being ingrained in healthcare, there are other ways to conceptualise health (Marvasti & Stafford, 2012). One important example is the World Health Organisation's definition of health as "complete physical, mental, and social wellbeing and not merely the absence of disease or infirmity" (WHO, 2022b). According to this definition, being healthy involves much more than not suffering from a disease or illness. This broader conceptualisation of health, championed by the WHO, not only challenges the traditional Western view but also offers an alternative perspective. It has driven the emergence of the construct of positive health, opening possibilities for a more comprehensive and proactive approach to wellbeing. The WHO also views health as "a resource for everyday life, not the objective of living", suggesting that health is an enabler of everyday life rather than an end in itself. Similarly, the WHO defines *mental health* as "a state of wellbeing in which every individual realises his or her own potential, can cope with the normal stresses of life, can work productively and fruitfully, and is able to make a contribution to her or his community" (WHO, 2022b). Let us explore the concept of mental health in more detail.

## MENTAL HEALTH

Expanding on the WHO conceptualisation of the mental health framework, Keyes and colleagues (2002) identified a significant knowledge gap in our understanding of mental health despite our comprehensive understanding of mental illness. To address this, a Mental Health Continuum (MHC) model was created that brought together the three leading conceptualisations of mental health: Psychological Wellbeing (Ryff, 1998), Subjective Wellbeing (Diener et al., 2018), and Social Wellbeing (Keyes, 1998. This revolutionary model reimagined mental health and mental illness as a continuum rather than a binary concept. As such, it categorised mental health into three distinct states: languishing, moderate health, and flourishing.

Experiencing languishing often feels like being in a limbo (Keyes, 2005). Individuals describe themselves as feeling empty, hollow, or stagnant when languishing. The "blah" feeling can be hard to shake off. Languishing can be more challenging to deal with than mental illness. It can be more frustrating than depression, as individuals may feel indifferent and lack a spark despite years of therapy, leading to a sense of giving up on themselves (Keyes et al., 2002). At the same time, languishing is different from mental illness.

When experiencing mental illness, people are more likely to actively seek help from health services, such as a GP or therapist, and they are more likely to receive a diagnosis and appropriate treatment. In contrast, those who languish may often not have enough symptoms of depression or anxiety to be diagnosed with it. At the same time, they report being less engaged in daily activities, less aware of their desires, and often miss some days at work. Languishing is a tricky state that often exists in a gap between mental illness and mental health. At the same time, it is essential to note that languishing can also occur concurrently with mental illness (Gilmour, 2014). Individuals who experienced a diagnosis with a mental health condition (e.g. depression; bipolar disorder; generalised anxiety disorder; alcohol, cannabis, or other drug abuse or dependence) over the previous 12 months, can also receive an optimal mental health diagnosis, although it is not common. As such, approximately 1% of languishers, 4.7% of moderately healthy individuals, and 4.5% of flourishers have been diagnosed with a mental health condition.

This suggests that, even though they are related, both conditions are relatively independent from each other and as such need to be addressed separately.

Individuals with moderate mental health often exhibit adequate levels of psychological wellbeing, as they regularly experience autonomy, personal growth, and self-acceptance. Moreover, they tend to encounter frequent positive emotional states, outnumbering negative emotions. This positive emotional landscape contributes to an overall sense of thriving. Importantly, they often have a supportive network of family and friends, enabling them to navigate life's complexities with greater ease and satisfaction. Together, these factors create a state of mental equilibrium, fostering moderate mental health.

Finally, some people experience a state of optimal wellbeing, i.e. flourishing. This state is associated with high levels of psychological, emotional, and social wellbeing, manifesting in their daily experiences. Research by Keyes et al. (2020) highlight the significance of flourishing in reducing the risk of major depressive episodes. Specifically, those who are languishing face a tenfold increase in risk, while individuals with moderate mental health see a sevenfold risk compared to their flourishing counterparts. Therefore, supporting people to experience flourishing will not only make them feel well but might also protect them from some mental health issues.

Flourishing is a significant contributor to a fulfilling life – a life filled with engagement, enriching relationships, and a sense of purpose. Importantly, it serves as a protective buffer against the onset of mental illness episodes. It empowers individuals to navigate life's challenges with resilience and grace, nurturing sustained mental and emotional wellness. At the same time, flourishing is a dynamic process; over a decade, 50% of flourishing individuals experienced a decline in wellbeing (Keyes, 2010). Similarly, those experiencing lower levels of wellbeing can flourish in the future. This gives us hope that many people who are currently on a languishing trajectory can change their direction by gaining knowledge and skills to flourish.

### Frank's story

*Frank has always been a happy person, full of energy and humour. Ever since he was at school, he made people laugh and was always the life of the party. At the same time, for the last few years, Frank has struggled with mental health issues, and was eventually diagnosed with bipolar disorder.*

*His mental health issues all began when Frank was in his early twenties. Feeling overwhelmed by the pressures of life, he turned to drugs as a way to cope. At first, it seemed to offer him an escape from his troubles, but soon enough, he found himself spiralling out of control. His moods became erratic, swinging from extreme highs to crushing lows. His family and friends had noticed a change in him. They offered a helping hand and he accepted.*

*In the midst of his struggles, Frank remained resilient. Through the support he received from his network, therapy and medication, he learned to manage his bipolar condition. But what surprised everyone was that despite all these challenges, Frank reported remarkably high levels of mental wellbeing. He had a clearly defined meaning in life – he was passionate about his work as an artist and found joy in spending time with his friends. He embraced himself fully, flaws and all, and had a deep self-acceptance, no matter what. All this helped him cope with his bipolar disorder, minimising the impact of his symptoms.*

*Frank's story is an example of how someone can grapple with a mental health condition while still learning to flourish. Despite the rollercoaster of emotions that bipolar disorder brought into his life, Frank found solace and fulfilment in the things that mattered most to him. His journey is an example of the complex interplay between mental illness and mental wellbeing, demonstrating that they can indeed coexist within the same person.*

## POSITIVE HEALTH

The concept of "positive health" has a rich and evolving history and has been a subject of intense debate for decades. While critics argue that existing definitions of health already encompass positive health states, proponents advocate for more precise definitions to enhance health outcomes, leading to a dynamic and ongoing discourse.

Positive health can be perceived from four distinct perspectives (Bodryzlova & Moullec, 2023), as illustrated in Figure 1.1. According to the first perspective, it is a one-dimensional concept deriving from positive psychology, which, similarly to the state of

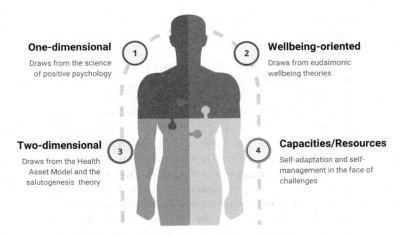

*Figure 1.1* Four conceptualisations of positive health.
Source: adapted from Bodryzlova & Moullec (2023).

flourishing, goes far beyond the mere absence of disease. It, therefore, encompasses various facets of wellbeing. Seligman (2008) states that it includes physical wellbeing, biological attributes, and functional perfection. Empirical studies have linked positive health to factors such as optimism, exercise, and quality of life in adults, while in children and adolescents, it is associated with good relationships, better cardiovascular fitness, healthy body weight, improved sleep quality, and positive behaviour (e.g. Padilla-Molledo et al., 2012).

The second perspective comes from Ryff and Singer (1998) who offer a significantly different viewpoint on positive health, positing it as more than mere absence of illness but a comprehensive state encompassing all aspects of individuals' lives. They delineate between eudaimonic wellbeing, which is centred on living a life of virtue and realising one's potential, vis-à-vis hedonic wellbeing, which focuses solely on happiness and life satisfaction. Their research suggests that positive health improves cardiovascular, neuroendocrine, and immune system functioning indicators. Subsequent to this debate by Ryff and Singer (2008) questionnaires have been developed to gauge various dimensions of wellbeing, including emotional, vocational, environmental, social, intellectual, physical, and spiritual aspects, as well as personal traits and interactive capabilities. Examples include the Salutogenic Wellness Promotion Scale (Becker et al., 2023) and the Psychological Wellbeing Scale (Ryff & Keyes, 1995), both showing inverse relationships with general health metrics and negative emotions.

The third perspective relates to the Health Assets Model (Bodryzlova et al., 2024), based on the Salutogenesis Theory (Vinje et al., 2007). It defines positive health as the ability to withstand adversities or maintain wellbeing even in their absence. It links individual characteristics with actions, environment and support available to them. This model highlights the importance of identifying and using existing personal assets to improve health outcomes, with a particular focus on resilience. This aspect is especially relevant in populations facing challenges, such as those experiencing childhood and adolescent cancer. By nurturing positive health in these contexts, not only are health outcomes improved, but also hope and resilience are fostered within individuals and communities.

The fourth perspective on positive health places a strong emphasis on capacities or resources that enable adaptation and self-management across physical, social, and emotional realms. This viewpoint highlights the importance of bodily and mental functions, quality of life, and social engagement. While the comprehensiveness of some models is debated, others have demonstrated reliability and validity in evaluating positive health. This conceptualisation aligns with broader notions of health as the cultivation of capabilities and personal resources that facilitate meaningful interaction with one's environment.

One example of the fourth perspective is a model developed in the Netherlands (Jung & van den Brekel-Dijskstra, 2021). It encourages patients to assess six aspects of their lives and then work on not only addressing their illness or disease but also explore their meaning in life, social networks and other concepts that make life worth living. These aspects include:

1. **Bodily Functions**: Patients assess their satisfaction with their physical health, including feeling healthy and fit, the presence of any complaints, quality of sleep, diet, and exercise habits.
2. **Mental Wellbeing**: This involves reflecting on their ability to communicate, their cheerfulness, self-acceptance, and sense of control.

3. **Meaning in Life**: Patients consider whether they accept their life, if their life has purpose and meaning, and whether they feel confident and grateful.
4. **Quality of Life**: This dimension includes feelings of health, safety, and happiness.
5. **Daily Functioning**: Patients evaluate their ability to take care of themselves, manage time and finances effectively.
6. **Participation**: This explores social contact, a sense of belonging, and support from others.

By working through each component, patients gain control over their own health and can make decisions about changes to improve their wellbeing. This approach extends beyond addressing the immediate physical or mental issues that prompted the visit, enabling GPs and other medical professionals to contribute to both treatment and prevention of diseases.

Adopting the positive health approach has proven effective, with a reported 25% reduction in hospital referrals from GP clinics, indicating its value in healthcare.

## RCSI PERSPECTIVE ON POSITIVE HEALTH

At RCSI University of Medicine and Health Sciences, we have developed a unique approach to positive health, offering distinct conceptualisations and pathways. Our approach aligns with other frameworks in recognising that the absence of illness does not equate to the presence of health, yet it also differs in other aspects.

While rooted in positive psychology research, our model extends its scope by incorporating both illness and disease alongside health and wellbeing. This broader perspective highlights that principles from positive psychology can be leveraged not only for prevention but also for reducing symptoms and potentially reversing some diseases. We address both eudaimonic aspects, such as personal growth or self-actualisation, and hedonic aspects of wellbeing, such as pleasure and comfort. This comprehensive approach, which acknowledges other models like Psychological Richness (Oishi & Westgate, 2021), enhances the resources and capabilities available for individuals to experience and maintain positive health.

Crucially, our application of positive health is non-prescriptive, empowering individuals to tailor their approach. We chose not to create models for applying positive health. Instead, we remain open to emerging concepts in positive psychology and related fields that can be adapted to health contexts. We encourage individuals to use all aspects of positive health according to their interests, values, and needs, testing and integrating a variety of activities to improve and maintain their positive health. This personalised approach that draws from what is best in positive psychology has the potential to guide people through their journey of the good life.

Lastly, our model uniquely combines the rapidly growing fields of positive psychology and lifestyle medicine. Positive psychology focuses on the science of wellbeing, while lifestyle medicine centres on preventing non-communicable diseases such as cancer, diabetes, and cardiovascular disease. This integration makes the RCSI perspective on positive health uniquely comprehensive, providing a solid foundation for understanding and promoting health.

We have extensively discussed our evolving understanding of positive health in previous works (Burke et al., 2023; O'Boyle et al., 2024). Here, we will focus on the primary characteristics of this paradigm. We have defined positive health as follows: "Positive health is both a destination and a journey. As a destination, it signifies the pinnacle of physical, mental, social, emotional, and meaningful thriving. As a journey, it reflects the fact that any movement towards thriving is a positive health journey" (O'Boyle et al., 2024). Similarly, Ryff and Singer (1998) describe positive health as "a multidimensional dynamic process rather than a discrete end state". Let's explore how this unfolds in real life.

### Anna's journey to positive health

*Anna had always been a hard worker, dedicated to her job as a marketing manager. However, she often felt stressed, tired, and disconnected from her friends and family. One day, after a particularly exhausting week, Anna decided it was time for a change. She wanted to feel better physically, mentally, emotionally, and socially. Thus, she began her journey towards positive health.*

*Anna started small, making gradual changes in her daily routine. She began by incorporating physical activity into her life. Initially, she* started with short walks in the park after work. As she felt more comfortable with physical activity, she joined a local gym and signed up to yoga classes. These activities improved her physical fitness and helped her manage stress and sleep better.

Next, Anna focused on her mental health. She started practising mindfulness meditation each morning, which helped her stay present and reduce anxiety. She also made time to read books she enjoyed and engage in creative activities like painting, which brought her joy and a sense of accomplishment.

Recognising the importance of social connections, Anna reached out to friends she had lost touch with. Initially, the meetings felt awkward, but soon, she was lost in engaging in conversations and forgot the initial jitters. She also expanded her social network by joining a community gardening club. These interactions enriched her social life gave her a feeling of a support system around her.

Anna has also begun to work on developing resilience. She attended therapy sessions to address long-standing issues and learn strategies to cope with life's ups and downs. She also found purpose in volunteering at a local animal shelter, which gave her a deeper sense of fulfilment and meaning.

Over time, Anna noticed that these small actions resulted in significant improvements in all areas of her life. She felt physically stronger, mentally clearer, socially connected, and emotionally balanced. Her life had become more meaningful, and she experienced a profound sense of thriving. This felt like an optimal state of wellbeing involving the body and mind. Or what they refer to at RCSI as positive health.

Anna also understood that this state was not a fixed endpoint. She realised that maintaining positive health required ongoing effort and adaptability. She continued to set new goals, like running a mini-marathon and learning a new language, ensuring that she kept moving forward on her journey.

Anna's story illustrates how positive health is a multidimensional dynamic process, a collection of small actions that result in profound outcomes. Each small step she took impacted other aspects of her health, creating a domino effect. Her physical activities boosted her mental health, her social interactions enhanced her emotional wellbeing, and her sense of purpose enriched every dimension of her life.

Anna's journey towards positive health demonstrates that it is both a destination and an ongoing process that matters. Reaching *the pinnacle of thriving involves continuous movement towards better physical, mental, social, emotional, and meaningful wellbeing. It is a dynamic and interconnected journey that requires ongoing commitment and adaptability.*

## THE CONTINUUM OF POSITIVE HEALTH

When considering our health, it is helpful to visualise ourselves along a continuum, ranging from severe illness (−10) to optimal wellbeing (+10) (see Figure 1.2). This framework draws from the insights of various scholars, including Antonovsky (1979, 1987, 1996), Ryff and Singer (1998), Seligman and Csikszentmihalyi (2000), Travis and Ryan (2004), and the WHO (2022a). A score of 0 indicates a state of absence of illness but not yet reaching peak functioning. While many of us may place ourselves somewhere to the right of 0 on this continuum when assessing our health, a few would rate themselves at a +10.

A particularly noteworthy state within this framework is languishing, characterised by a lack of mental health despite the absence of illness. During languishing, individuals experience dissatisfaction, struggle to engage, and find their interests diminished (Keyes et al., 2002). This condition became more apparent for many during the COVID-19 pandemic.

Traditionally, health services have been oriented toward treating illness and disease, focusing primarily on the 0 to −10 range of the spectrum. Goals typically continue to revolve around curing the patient, preventing further decline, or maintaining quality of life in the face of stable deterioration. While preventive and public health medicine aims to prevent illness and disease, the disease model often influences their objectives.

A more holistic approach to health encompasses treatment and prevention, extending its focus to the 0 to +10 range of the continuum. This broader perspective acknowledges the interconnectedness between individual health and the environment, recognising that both influence individuals' position and trajectory along the continuum (Figure 1.2).

Positive health presents a departure from the prevalent approach that defines health solely in terms of the absence of illness and disease (Ickovics & Park, 1998; Ryff & Singer, 1998). It aims to

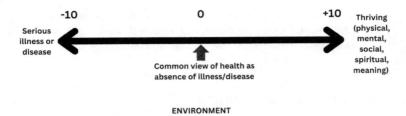

*Figure 1.2* Model of positive health.

Source: authors.

redirect focus and resources towards enhancing health and wellbeing for individuals coping with illness and those not. While formulations of positive health have been proposed previously (Bodryzlova & Moullec, 2023), their adoption has been gradual. Recent interest in the positive health framework is influenced by several factors. Figure 1.3 explores them in more detail.

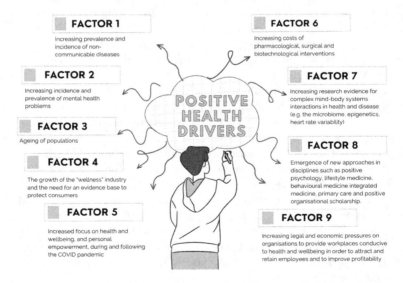

*Figure 1.3* Factors driving the emergence of the scientific positive health paradigm.

Source: For a more detailed discussion see O'Boyle et al. (2024, pp. 2–23).

## TEN PRINCIPLES OF POSITIVE HEALTH

1. Positive health is a philosophical rather than a purely medical concept. Here, the philosophical tradition of understanding "the goods in life" (having a purpose, having good social connections, having good self-regard and having a sense of mastery) are essential dimensions of positive health.

2. Health is not (merely) the absence of disease or illness; the absence of mental or physical conditions does not ensure positive health.

3. Positive health is not a static destination but a dynamic journey. It is not solely about reaching a desired end state but also about the progress made towards thriving, irrespective of one's current health status. It's not just about where one is on the spectrum, but also the direction they are facing and the pace at which they are moving along it.

4. Positive health is a multidimensional construct involving physical, emotional, social, and meaningful functioning. Individuals may be at different points regarding these components at any given time.

5. Positive health is not merely about empowering individuals to optimise their lives owing to the impact of an individual's environment and the potential for environmental factors to positively or negatively impact health.

6. Positive health is desirable in its own right, but it has also been shown to buffer against mental and physical illness.

7. Emerging research on the ubiquity and intricacy of complex mind–body interactions highlights the need for holistic, systemic approaches to positive health. Minds, brains, and bodies are closely intertwined and mutually interdependent. The physiological bases of thriving may be unique and may not simply mirror pathological processes. This call for a holistic approach empowers healthcare professionals to consider all aspects of an individual's health in their practice.

8. Positive health interventions are not exclusive to a particular group; they are relevant for everyone, both ill and well.

The aim is to move people or help them move themselves to the right on the continuum, no matter what their starting point. This inclusivity highlights the importance of each individual's journey towards positive health.

9. Health services have evolved largely to treat disease and illness rather than enhance health in the sense that the term is used in positive health. Improving health requires a systems approach focusing on individual, collective, and environmental factors.

10. Positive health is relevant for everyone: those who have an illness, disease, or disability and those who do not.

## DISCIPLINES RELATED TO POSITIVE HEALTH

### LIFESTYLE MEDICINE

Lifestyle medicine is currently considered the most rapidly growing medical field committed to preventing, managing, alleviating, and potentially reversing non-communicable diseases like diabetes, cancer, and cardiovascular ailments. These diseases, are significant global contributors to premature deaths and have therefore become a pressing global health issue. Lifestyle medicine approach involves advocating for whole food plant-based diets, physical activity, sleeping well, effective stress management strategies, discouraging harmful substance use, and fostering social networks (Frates et al., 2019). These six pillars of lifestyle medicine are illustrated in Figure 1.4.

### POSITIVE PSYCHOLOGY

Positive psychology is a science of wellbeing and optimal human functioning (Burke, 2022). It began as an exploration of what is right, rather than wrong, with human beings and their daily life experiences. By 1998, the ratio of research on happiness versus depression was 1:17 (Achor, 2011). This meant our knowledge about wellbeing was negatively skewed, and that imbalance needed to be addressed urgently. Year after year, more research was

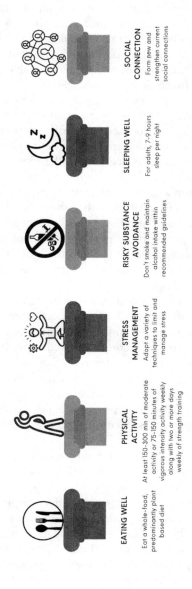

*Figure 1.4* The six pillars of lifestyle medicine.

Source: Adapted from *The Pillar Booklet*. American College of lifestyle medicine. https://lifestylemedicine.org/wp-content/uploads/2022/07/Pillar-Booklet.pdf

conducted about the positive aspects of the human experience. For example, within leadership practice, over a decade the number of academic articles published increased from 2% to 10% (Rusk & Waters, 2013), thus the objective of the initial call for research on positive traits, positive experiences and positive organisations, institutions and communities (Seligman & Csikszentmihalyi, 2000) has effectively changed the psychological landscape.

The second wave of positive psychology came about in response to researchers and practitioners misunderstanding the first wave of positive psychology as a field focused primarily on positive traits and experiences without considering the benefits of the negative. True wellbeing comes from negotiating the tension between opposite forces influencing each other, ying and yang, the good and the bad, the optimism and the pessimism, or happiness and suffering (Lomas & Ivtzan, 2016). Within this wave it is claimed you can't have one without the other. Thus, positive psychology is not about focusing on developing those positive aspects of the human psyche but embracing the good, the bad and the ugly and figuring out how the knowledge of both can help us grow and become the foundation for our wellbeing.

Finally, the third wave of positive psychology emerged to advocate for more complexity (Lomas et al., 2020). It encouraged expanding the knowledge and skills to go beyond the individual by considering the systems and other factors impacting their wellbeing. It called for interdisciplinary and multicultural explorations that embrace various research methodologies to help us understand the concepts better. The third wave of positive psychology, while embracing complexity, also acknowledges the challenges it presents, highlighting the need for continuous exploration and adaptation. This is also the wave that gave rise to positive health.

Positive health is a natural progression where positive psychology intersects with lifestyle medicine (Lianov, 2019). The rationale for it is deeply rooted in the many overlapping concepts within each field. For instance, research indicates that positive affective processes can drive positive behaviour change, enhancing adherence to healthy behaviours by making them more salient and triggering unconscious motivation for those behaviours (Linaov, 2024). At the same time, positive emotions can also directly impact physical health (van Cappellen et al., 2018). Increased positive emotions lead to increases in vagal tone mediated by social interactions (Kok et al., 2013). Therefore, the fusion of these two fields of research is a logical and necessary step that will enhance both fields.

---

Our research at the RCSI Centre for positive health Sciences in Ireland showed some practical insights into the connection between lifestyle medicine and psychological flourishing. Individuals experiencing psychological flourishing were nine times more likely to incorporate at least three pillars of lifestyle medicine into their routine, such as regular walks, healthy eating habits, or quality sleep, than those experiencing languishing. This means that by adopting these lifestyle factors, individuals may significantly enhance their psychological, emotional, and social wellbeing. This study provides the first evidence of a correlation between the pursuit of preventing non-communicable diseases and achieving optimal levels of wellbeing. It offer a tangible path towards living a healthier and happier life. For further details, go to Burke and Dunne (2023).

---

## HEALTH PSYCHOLOGY

Health Psychology, a subset of psychology, that applies psychological theories and principles to health, illness, and healthcare (for a review, see Marks et al., 2020; Ogden, 2023). Health psychology's focus on the determinants of behavioural change adds great value to positive health. For instance, models, such as the Transtheoretical Model of Change (Prochaska et al., 2007) and the emerging practice of positive health coaching (Frates et al., 2019; Van Nieuwerburg & Knight, 2024) offer significant insights into pathways for fostering personal transformation. RCSI's positive health approach is informed by behaviour change models and other research within the realm of health psychology relating to the positive aspects of human experiences.

## SALUTOGENESIS

Salutogenesis, heavily influencing the construct of positive health, stems from the framework developed by Aaron Antonovsky (Antonovsky,

1979, 1996). Antonovsky coined a new term, "salutogenesis", to refer to the factors that drive health, in contrast to the term "pathogenesis" which refers to the factors that drive illness and disease. Rather than health and illness being seen as binary phenomena, he postulated that everyone is on a continuum from "dis-ease" to "ease". The key question for Antonovsky was what are the factors that move a person in the direction of "ease", i.e. the factors that make people healthy, and he proposed that such an approach would be more productive as a framework for research (Antonovsky, 1979, 1987, 1996; Mittlemark et al, 2022).

A particular focus of salutogenesis in the extent to which an individual possesses health assets which allow them to resist adversity or maintain wellbeing and this has been a key influence on the positive health construct. Antonovsky proposed that a key a psychological orientation, called by him the sense of coherence – the extent to which one has a pervasive, enduring feeling of confidence that one's internal and external environments are predictable and that there is a high probability that things will work out well – was particularly important for health and wellbeing (Antonovsky, 1979, 1987). This conceptualisation has influenced thinking in positive health research, and it has been proposed that positive health can be defined in terms of capacities or resources, such as the ability to adapt and manage oneself in the face of challenges across physical, social, and emotional domains. This perspective emphasises bodily and mental functions, quality of life and social participation. Although there are concerns about the comprehensiveness of models such as this, there is some evidence for the reliability and validity of resource type measures in assessing positive health (Bodryzlova and Moullec, 2023) This conceptualisation aligns with broader views of health as the development of capabilities and personal resources that enable meaningful functioning and interaction with one's environment.

## ARE THE BIOLOGICAL SUBSTRATES OF POSITIVE HEALTH DIFFERENT FROM THOSE OF DISEASE?

Understanding the structure and functioning of the body through such disciplines as anatomy, physiology and biochemistry is the cornerstone of modern healthcare. In medicine, the main concern is understanding the processes by which things go wrong and this has led to the emergence of major disciplines such as pathology and microbiology. Modern medical science has provided a huge body of knowledge about the disease processes, trauma and ageing. The emerging positive health paradigm offers an intriguing challenge to determine what the biological substrates for wellbeing might be (Cloninger, 2012). It may be that the mechanisms underlying thriving are unique and may not mirror those of disease (Ryff et al., 2004; Seals et al., 2015). How, for example, are we to understand the link between an optimistic mindset and decreased mortality (Lee et al., 2019) or the relationship between a sense of coherence and biological markers of health (Lindfors et al., 2005)?

A study involving over 6,000 participants in the United Kingdom was conducted as part of the Health and Lifestyle Survey, spanning nearly a decade. Researchers asked participants about symptoms of ill-being, such as alcoholism, and symptoms of wellbeing, including a sense of meaning in life and experiencing positive emotions. For many participants, mental illness was negatively correlated with mental health, indicating that as they experienced mental illness, they also reported reduced levels of mental health. However, over 30% of participants exhibited both higher levels of mental illness and higher levels of mental health. This study demonstrated that mental illness and mental health can be independent of each other. Therefore, focusing solely on reducing mental illness is not enough to promote good mental health. To read more, go to Huppert and Whittington (2003).

Exciting new possibilities for understanding wholistic health are now emerging, showing intricate systemic interactions, such as those between the gut and the brain (Cryan et al., 2019), genetic expression and cognition, and emotion (Feinberg, 2008), as well as psychological processes and immune function (Kusnecov & Anisman,

2014). Research relating to positive affect offers intriguing evidence of an interplay between positive states and the neurobiological substrates of information processing (Garland et al., 2010). This type of research is opening the door to new ways of understanding how we function and the possibility exists that we will discover new mechanisms which we have missed in the past because of our overriding focus on pathological processes.

## POSITIVE HEALTH INTERVENTIONS

What distinguishes the RCSI positive health Centre's approach from others is its extensive range of interventions designed to enhance positive health. positive health Interventions (PHIs) are defined as "tools that aim to build psychological, emotional, intellectual, physiological, and social resources, demonstrating evidence of improving health and wellbeing, and reducing the burden of disease" (Burke et al., 2024, p. 193). These tools integrate positive psychology and lifestyle medicine techniques, showing evidence of (1) positive outcomes, including psychological benefits like flourishing, self-esteem, optimism, and positive affect, as well as physiological benefits like heart-rate variability, cortisol levels, and intestinal permeability, and (2) symptom reduction in both mental and physical health contexts (Burke et al., 2023).

Burke et al. (2023) have created a comprehensive collection of over 100 research-based tools that fit the definition of positive health Interventions. They proposed these tools can either continuously build resources or serve as interventions during challenging times. However, they also stressed the importance of selecting tools that resonated personally with individuals, and integrating them into existing wellbeing practices rather than replacing any current approaches. Furthermore, they encouraged an open mind when practising them and varying activities to avoid boredom. They also advocated for practising the tools with others, such as friends and family members, and going on a positive health journey with them.

The tools are categorised into eight distinct groups, with examples provided in Table 1.1.

This list of PHIs is not exhaustive, as many more activities continue to be included as long as they demonstrate evidence of promoting

*Table 1.1* Example of positive health interventions (tools)

| Category | Examples of tools |
| --- | --- |
| Calming | Sleep, Meditation, Nature, Creativity, Green care |
| Energising | Physical activity, Nutrition, Play, Humour |
| Coping | Expressive writing, Optimism, Bibliotherapy, Stress mindset, Compassion |
| Feeling good | Reminiscing, Strengths, Gratitude, Music, Art viewing |
| Meaning making | Exploring meaning, Positive identity, Benefit finding, Legacy, Photography |
| Relationships | Capitalisation, Forgiveness, Kindness, Savouring, |
| Prospecting | Anticipation, Goals setting, Best possible self, Hope, |
| Emerging | Storytelling, Self-care, Social media diet, Self-reassurance |

Source: Burke, J., Dunne, P.J., Meehan, T., O'Boyle, C.A., Van Nieuwerburgh, C. (2023). *Positive health: 100+ research-based positive psychology and lifestyle medicine tools to enhance your wellbeing.* Routledge.

physiological and psychological wellbeing and supporting individuals in managing illness and disease symptoms. Recently, Burke and Dunne (2024) examined the effects of lifestyle medicine tools vis-à-vis the combination of lifestyle medicine and positive psychology tools. We found that while there were some improvements in wellbeing, the tools had an adverse impact on participants' sleep. Therefore, it is essential to monitor the impact of wellbeing tools on health, and further research is needed to explore this topic in greater depth.

Furthermore, Lianov and Burke (2024) recently explored the integration of positive psychology within lifestyle medicine. Their focus was on exploring ways in which medical professionals could use positive psychology and lifestyle medicine in their practice. To do so, the authors reviewed extensively the latest literature in positive psychology as it pertained to each pillar of lifestyle medicine. Additionally, they examined a variety of positive health interventions applicable in clinical practice. Their book presented positive psychology research as a means to enhance the effectiveness of lifestyle medicine practice, offering practical examples of applying positive health in medicine that are within reach of every medical professional.

## POSITIVE HEALTH COACHING

Positive health Coaching model, as developed by van Nieuwerburgh and Knight (2024), represents a fresh approach to coaching that incorporates the concept of positive health. It is "a managed conversational process that supports individuals in achieving meaningful goals while enhancing their wellbeing". In this coaching model, equal emphasis is placed on both goal attainment and wellbeing. The approach comprises four essential components:

1. It involves a set of partnership principles designed to cultivate respectful and empowering relationships.
2. It requires the use of highly developed conversational skills to facilitate empowering dialogues.
3. It uses a powerful conversational framework grounded in the elements of the Impact Cycle (Identify–Learn–Improve).
4. It adopts a dialogical approach that facilitates a confident and transparent knowledge exchange between and coach and a client.

Despite being in its early stages of development, this innovative coaching method, drawing from evidence-based practices in positive psychology, health psychology, and coaching, shows significant potential.

## SUMMARY

Positive health has emerged as a new way of thinking about health and illness in recent years. Those who support this approach aim to challenge the common belief that health only means being free from disease. They also advocate for a health framework that applies to everyone, regardless of their current health status or susceptibility to illness. This inclusive approach has important implications for the future of medicine. The rise of personalised medicine is an example of this shift, emphasising disease prevention and health promotion over traditional bio-medical treatment methods. The International Consortium for Personalised Medicine predicts a transformative change in healthcare priorities by 2030, focusing on assessing risks, categorising patients, and using personalised strategies for health promotion and disease prevention – especially important for aging populations (Vincente et al., 2020).

One of the main challenges with the concept of positive health is the risk of placing too much emphasis on individual responsibility for health outcomes. It is essential to acknowledge that environmental factors play a significant role in shaping health. The World Health Organisation recognizes genetics, social circumstances, environmental exposures, behavioral patterns, and access to healthcare as influential determinants of health (WHO, 2021). The COVID-19 pandemic has highlighted the importance of addressing both individual health behaviours and the broader systemic factors that affect health outcomes. Therefore, experiencing positive health requires a holistic approach that takes into account both individual actions, environmental influences and interconnecting relationships.

## REFERENCES

Achor, S. (2011). *The happiness advantage: The seven principles of positive psychology that fuel success and performance at work.* Virgin Books.

Antonovsky, A. (1979). *Health, stress and coping.* Jossey-Bass.

Antonovsky, A. (1987). *Unravelling the mystery of health: How people manage stress and stay well.* Jossey-Bass.

Antonovsky, A. (1996). The salutogenic model as a theory to guide health promotion. *Health Promotion International, 11*, 11–18.

Becker, C. M., Bian, H., Martin, R. J., Sewell, K., Stellefson, M., & Chaney, B. (2023). Development and field test of the Salutogenic Wellness Promotion Scale – short form (SWPS-SF) in U.S. college students. *Global Health Promotion, 30*(1), 16–22. https://doi.org/10.1177/17579759221102193

Bodryzlova, Y., & Moullec, G. (2023). Definitions of Positive Health: A systematic scoping review. *Global Health Promotion*, *30*(3), 6–14. https://doi.org/10.1177/17579759221139802

Bodryzlova, Y., Moullec, G., & Kelly, M. P. (2024). The Dynamic Model of Health Assets: A model development. *Global Health Promotion*, *0*(0). https://doi.org/10.1177/17579759241248624

Bonniwell, I. (2024). Positive psychology breakthroughs. In J. Burke, I. Boniwell, B. Frates, L. S. Liana, & C. A. O'Boyle (Eds.). *Routledge international handbook of positive health sciences*. Routledge.

Bonniwell, I., & Tunariu, A. D. (2019). *Positive psychology: Theory, research and applications* (2nd ed). Open University Press.

Burke, J., & Dunne, P. J. (2024). Mind meets body: Lifestyle medicine and positive psychology interventions for school. In G. Arslan & M. Yildirim (Eds.), *Handbook of positive school psychology interventions: Evidence-based practice for promoting youth mental health*. Springer.

Burke, J., Dunne, P. J., Meehan, T., O'Boyle, C. A., Van Nieuwerburgh, C. (2023). *Positive health: 100+ research-based positive psychology and lifestyle medicine tools to enhance your wellbeing*. Routledge.

Burke, J., Boniwell, I., Frates, B., Lianov, L. S., O'Boyle, C. A. (2024). *Routledge international handbook of Positive Health sciences*. Routledge.

Cloninger, C. R., Salloum, I. M., & Mezzich, J. E. (2012). The dynamic origins of health and wellbeing. *International Journal Person Centred Medicine*, *2*(2), 179–187. https://doi.org/10.5750/ijpcm.v2i2.213

Cryan, J. F., O'Riordan, K. J., Cowan, C. S. M., Sandhu, K. V., Bastiaanssen, T. F. S., Boehme, M., Codagnone, M. G., Cussotto, S. … Dinan, T. G. (2019). The Microbiota-Gut-Brain Axis. *Physiological Review*, *99*(4), 1877–2013. https://doi.org/10.1152/physrev.00018.2018

Diener, E., Oishi, S., & Tay, L. (2018). Advances in subjective well-being research. *Nature Human Behaviour*, *2*(4), 253–260. https://doi.org/10.1038/s41562-018-0307-6

Engel, G. L. (1977). The need for a new medical model: A challenge for biomedicine. *Science*, *196*, 129–135.

Feinberg, A. P. (2008). Epigenetics at the epicenter of modern medicine. *JAMA*, *299*(11), 1345–1350. https://doi.org/10.1001/jama.299.11.1345

Frates, B., Bonnet, J. P., Joseph, R., & Peterson, J. A. (2019). *The lifestyle medicine handbook: An introduction to the power of healthy habits*. Healthy Learning.

Garland, E. L., Fredrickson, B., Kring, A. M., Johnson, D. P., Meyer, P. S., Penn, D. L. (2010). Upward spirals of positive emotions counter downward spirals of negativity: Insights from the broaden-and-build theory and affective neuroscience on the treatment of emotion dysfunctions and deficits inbpsychopathology. *Clinical Psychology Review*, *30*(7), 849–864.

Gilmour, H. (2014). Positive mental health and mental illness. *Health Reports*, *25*, 3–9.

Huppert, F. A., & Whittington, J. E. (2003). Evidence for the independence of positive and negative wellbeing: Implications for quality of life assessment. *British Journal of Health Psychology*, *8*, 107–122.

Ickovics, J. R., & Park, C. L. (1998). Paradigm shift: Why a focus on health is important. *Journal of Social Issues*, *54*(2), 237–244.

Jung, H. P., & van den Brekel-Dijskstra, K. (2021). *Handbook of positive health in primary care*. Bohn Stafleu van Loghum.

Keyes, C. L. M. (1998). Social well-being. *Social Psychology Quarterly*, *61*(2), 121–140. https://doi.org/10.2307/2787065

Keyes, C. L. M. (2005). Mental illness and/or mental health? Investigating axioms of the complete state model of health. *Journal of Consulting and Clinical Psychology*, *73*, 539–548.

Keyes, C. L., Shmotkin, D., & Ryff, C. D. (2002). Optimizing wellbeing: The empirical encounter of two traditions. *Journal of Personality and Social Psychology*, *82*(6), 1007–1022.

Keyes, C. L. (2010). The next steps in the promotion and protection of positive mental health. *Canadian Journal of Nursing Research*, *42*(3), 17–28.

Keyes, C. L. M., Yao, J., Hybels, C. F., Milstein, G., & Proeschold-Bell, R. J. (2020). Are changes in positive mental health associated with increased likelihood of depression over a two year period? A test of the mental health promotion and protection hypotheses. *Journal of Affective Disorders*, *270*, 136–142. https://doi.org/10.1016/j.jad.2020.03.056

Kok, B. E., Coffey, K. A., Cohn, M. A., Catalino, L. I., Vacharkulksemsuk, T., Algoe, S. B., Brantley, M., & Fredrickson, B. L. (2013). How positive emotions build physical health: Perceived positive social connections account for for the upward spiral between positive emotions and vagal tone. *Psychological Science*, *24*, 1123–1132.

Kusnecov, A.W., & Anisman, H. (2014). *The Wiley-Blackwell handbook of psychoneuroimmunology*. John Wiley.

Lai, A. G., & Chang, W. H. (2022). There is no health without mental health: Challenges ignored and lessons learned. *Clinical and Translational Medicine*, *12*(6), e897. https://doi.org/10.1002/ctm2.897

Lee, L. O., James, P., Zevon, E. S., Kim, E. S., Trudel-Fitzgerald, C., Spiro, A., Grodstein, F., & Kubzansky, L. D. (2019). Optimism is associated with exceptional longevity in 2 epidemiologic cohorts of men and women. *Proceedings of the National Academy of Sciences of the United States of America*, *116*(37), 18357–18362. https://doi.org/10.1073/pnas.1900712116

Leonardi, F. (2018). The definition of health: Towards new perspectives. *International Journal of Health Services*, *48*(4), 735–748. https://doi.org/10.1177/0020731418782653

Lianov, L. S. (2019). *Roots of positive change: Optimizing health care with positive psychology*. American College of Lifestyle Medicine.

Lianov, L. S. (2024). Applying positive psychology and the pillars of lifestyle medicine. In J. Burke, B. Boniwell, B. Frates, L. S. Lianov, C. A. O'Boyle (Eds.), *Routledge international handbook of Positive Health sciences* (pp. 314–319). Routledge.

Lianov, L., & Burke, J. (2024). *Lifestyle medicine inside and out: A guide on how to apply positive psychology in person-centred medicine*. Routledge.

Lindfors, P., Lundberg, O., & Lundberg, U. (2005). Sense of coherence and biomarkers of health in 43 year old women. *International Journal of Behavioural Medicine, 12*(2), 98–102.

Lomas, T., & Ivtzan, I. (2016). Second wave positive psychology: Exploring the positive–negative dialectics of wellbeing. *Journal of Happiness Studies: An Interdisciplinary Forum on Subjective Well-Being, 17*(4), 1753–1768. https://doi.org/10.1007/s10902-015-9668-y

Lomas, T., Waters, L., Williams, P., Oades, L., & Kern, M. (2020). Third wave positive psychology: Broadening towards complexity. *Journal of Positive Psychology, 16*. https://doi.org/10.1080/17439760.2020.1805501

Marks, D. F., Murray, M., & Estacio, E. V. (2020). *Health psychology: Theory, research and practice*. Sage.

Marvasti, F. F., & Stafford, R. S. (2012). From sick care to health care: Reengineering prevention into the U.S. system. *New England Journal of Medicine, 367* (10), 889–891.

Mittelmark, M. B., Bauer, G. F., Vaandrager, L., Pelikan, J. M., Sagy, S., Eriksson, M., Lindstrom, B., & Meier Magistretti, C. (2022). *The handbook of salutogenesis* (2nd ed.). Springer International. https://doi.org/10.1007/978-3-030-79515-3

O'Boyle, C. A., Lianov, L., Burke, J., Frates, B., & Boniwell, I. (2024). Positive health: An emerging new construct. In J. Burke, I. Boniwell, B. Frates, L. S. Lianov, C. A. O'Boyle (Eds.), *Routledge international handbook of Positive Health sciences* (pp. 2–23). Routledge.

Oishi, S., & Westgate, E. C. (2021). A psychologically rich life: Beyond happiness and meaning. *Psychological Review, 129*(4), 790–811. http://dx.doi.org/10.1037/rev0000317

Ogden, J. (2023). *Health psychology* (7th ed.). McGraw-Hill.

Padilla-Moledo, C., Castro-Piñero, J., Ortega, F. B., Mora, J., Márquez, S., Sjöström, M., Ruiz, J. R. (2012). Positive health, cardiorespiratory fitness and fatness in children and adolescents, *European Journal of Public Health, 22*(1), 52–56, https://doi.org/10.1093/eurpub/ckr005

Prochaska, J. O., Norcross, J. C., & DiClemente, C. C. (2007). *Changing for good*. William Morrow.

Rusk, R. D., & Waters, L. E. (2013). Tracing the size, reach, impact, and breadth of positive psychology. *Journal of Positive Psychology, 8*(3), 207–221. https://doi.org/10.1080/17439760.2013.777766

Ryff, C. D., & Keyes, C. L. M. (1995). The structure of psychological well-being revisited. *Journal of Personality and Social Psychology, 69*(4), 719–727.

Ryff, C. D., & Singer, B. (1998). The contours of positive human health. *Psychological Inquiry, 9*(1), 1–28. https://doi.org/10.1207/s15327965pli 0901_1

Ryff, C. D., Singer, B. H., & Dienberg Love, G. (2004). Positive health: Connecting wellbeing with biology. *Philosophical transactions of the Royal Society of London. Series B, Biological sciences, 359*(1449), 1383–1394. https://doi.org/10.1098/rstb.2004.1521

Seals, D. R., Justice, J. N., & LaRocca, T. J. (2016). Physiological geroscience: Targeting function to increase healthspan and achieve optimal longevity. *Journal of Physiology, 594*(8), 2001–2024. https://doi.org/10.1113/jphysiol.2014.282665

Seligman, M. E. P. (2008). Positive Health. *Applied Psychology: An International Review, 57,* 3–18. https://doi.org/10.1111/j.1464-0597.2008.00351.x

Seligman, M. E. P., & Csikszentmihalyi, M. (2000). Positive psychology: An introduction. *American Psychologist, 55*(1) 5–14.

Travis, J. W., & Ryan, R. S. (2004). *The wellness workbook: How to achieve enduring health and vitality* (3rd ed.). Celestial Arts.

van Capellan, P., Rice, E. L., Catalino, L. I., & Fredrickson, B. L. (2018). Positive affective processes underlie Positive Health behaviour change. *Psychological Health, 33*(1), 77–97. https://doi.org/10.1080/08870446.2017.1320798

Van Nieuwerburg, C., & Knight, J. (2024). Positive health coaching: Adopting a dialogical approach to health and wellbeing. In J. Burke, I. Boniwell, B. Frates, L. S. Lianov, & C. A. O'Boyle (Eds.), *Routledge international handbook of Positive Health sciences* (pp. 220–237). Routledge.

Vicente, A. M., Ballensiefen, W., & Jönsson, J. I. (2020). How personalised medicine will transform healthcare by 2030: The ICPerMed vision. *Journal of Translational Medicine, 18*(1), 180. https://doi.org/10.1186/s12967-020-02316-w

Vinje, H. F., Langeland, E., Bull, T. (2016). Aaron Antonovsky's development of salutogenesis, 1979 to 1994. In M. B. Mittelmark, S. Sagy, M. Eriksson et al. (Eds.), *The Handbook of Salutogenesis* [Internet]. Springer, chapter 4. www.ncbi.nlm.nih.gov/books/NBK435860/ doi: 10.1007/978-3-319-04600-6_4

World Health Organization (2021). *Social determinants of health.* www.who.int/health-topics/social-determinants-of-health#tab=tab_1

World Health Organization (2022a). *World mental health report: Transforming mental health for all.* www.who.int/teams/mental-health-and-substance-use/world-mental-health-report

World Health Organization (2022b). *Basic documents 49th edition. Constitution.* https://apps.who.int/gb/bd/pdf_files/BD_49th-en.pdf#page=6

# 2

# POSITIVE MENTAL HEALTH

One of the most critical aspects of the positive health approach is its recognition that anyone, regardless of their health status, can experience the highest levels of wellbeing, known as psychological flourishing. Let us begin this chapter by delving into the existing wellbeing models that can serve as practical guides for individuals on their pathway to flourishing. Then, we will explore how individuals can combine the fields of lifestyle medicine and positive psychology to create the science of positive health. Finally, we will explore ways in which they can apply it in their real life.

### Maggie's and Sarah's journey

*Maggie and Sarah have been best friends since childhood, sharing countless adventures and a mutual love for fun. They laughed together, supported each other, and shared dreams of living fulfilling lives. Despite their similarities, they discovered something incredible when they began working with a health coach: the things that made their lives truly worthwhile were quite different.*

*Maggie thrived on excitement and pleasure. Her days were filled with spontaneous road trips, lively parties, and new experiences that invigorated her. She believed in living in the moment, soaking up joy wherever possible. For Maggie, a worthwhile life was full of fun and excitement, where happiness was found in the thrill of the here and now.*

*While equally enthusiastic about fun, Sarah deeply longed for authenticity and purpose. She sought a life that was not only enjoyable but also meaningful. Sarah wanted her actions to align with her*

DOI: 10.4324/9781003457169-2

values and beliefs, ensuring her life had a clear direction and purpose. She believed that true fulfilment came from living authentically, making choices that reflected her true self, and contributing to something greater than herself.

When both friends decided to gain healthy weight, they approached a positive health coach for guidance. As they delved into different models of wellbeing, their distinct ways of thinking and being became even more apparent. The health coach, recognising their unique needs, helped them design personalised pathways to achieve their goals.

For Maggie, the focus was on integrating fun and enjoyment into her health journey and those "aha" moments that helped her grow psychologically. Her plan included engaging in activities such as dance classes, new cuisine cooking for her house parties, and sports that she loved and put a smile on her face. Maggie's health plan was designed to ensure that every step towards gaining a healthy weight was filled with pleasure and excitement, making the process enjoyable and sustainable for her.

On the other hand, Sarah's approach was rooted in her quest for authenticity and purpose. Her plan involved activities that resonated with her values, such as mindful eating, yoga, the Buddhist way of thinking behind it, and volunteering at the homeless shelter. Sarah wanted to ensure that her journey towards a healthier weight was not just about physical changes but also about aligning with her deeper sense of purpose in life. Her health plan was carefully designed to reflect her authentic self and desire for a meaningful life.

As they progressed, Maggie and Sarah's bond grew stronger as friends, each celebrating the other's milestones. Maggie would eagerly share her latest fun recipes, while Sarah would speak proudly about the fulfilment she found in her volunteer work. They laughed together, encouraged each other, and respected their different paths, yet the outcome for both was the same, happy with their lives and the people they became after years of senseless diets, which left them undernourished.

Through the process of positive health coaching, Maggie and Sarah discovered that their definitions of a fulfilling life were unique. Yet, both friends, despite their different paths, were able to achieve their health goals as planned.

Four main wellbeing approaches exist, referred to as flourishing models in positive psychology that inform positive health. Most of them are derived from two distinct philosophical perspectives: hedonic and eudaimonic. Hedonic wellbeing relates to wellbeing gained by pursuing pleasure and happiness, encapsulated in the psychological subjective wellbeing model (Diener, 1985). This model includes emotional experiences (affect) and life satisfaction. Research shows that happiness, or hedonic wellbeing, is associated with experiencing more positive than negative emotions, highlighting the balance between the two. Life satisfaction, the second component, reflects a cognitive aspect of happiness. As such, the hedonic wellbeing approach is one of the most frequently quoted approaches to measuring especially large-scale wellbeing. For example, the famous "World Happiness Report" is based on the concept of hedonic wellbeing, although increasingly, the researchers use eudaimonic aspects of it too.

---

### INTENSELY POSITIVE EXPERIENCES

#### (Adapted from Burton & King, 2004)

Think about some of the happiest moments in your life – those times that filled your heart with pure joy. This could be when you fell in love, when your baby was born, when you were moved by a piece of music or another unforgettable experience. Choose one memory and spend the next 15–20 minutes writing about it in as much detail as possible. Don't worry about mistakes, spelling, or grammar. Instead, focus on your thoughts, feelings, emotions, circumstances, the people around you, and everything that made that moment special. Let yourself relive the positive emotions this happy memory brought you.

---

Hedonic wellbeing, with its nuanced association with lifestyle medicine, is a complex perspective on positive health. For instance, a study with young people found that soft drink consumption was associated with a higher risk of being overweight but also with increased happiness (Lin et al., 2023). Another research demonstrated an inverted U-shaped relationship between happiness and obesity, whereby being underweight or obese was linked to unhappiness (Liu et al., 2022). The happiest people's weight was moderate. Let us stop and consider the implications of these studies. On the one hand, they show that consuming unhealthy products could give people a boost of pleasurable emotions, thus facilitating happiness. As such, removing the unhealthy product, e.g. a soft drink, could make us healthier but potentially less happy. This is why, before individuals replace soft drinks and other unhealthy products with healthier ones, exploring ways to find pleasure from other sources may be useful. This way, their risk of reduced happiness will be lowered. At the same time, having moderate weight makes individuals the happiest compared to those at either end of this continuum. Weight management plays a crucial role in maintaining positive emotions, as it can prevent weight-related issues from becoming a source of unhappiness. Not having to cope with these sources of unhappiness could help us maintain higher positive emotions, improving our overall happiness. These are just two examples of the complex relationship between happiness and lifestyle medicine. Throughout this book, we will explore other examples.

---

### MUSIC

#### (Majeed et al., 2021)

For 30 minutes before going to bed, listen to music – whatever tune you like. In a study, individuals who listened to music every night before bed for ten weeks reported better sleep quality, more significant stress decline, and improved subjective wellbeing when assessed in the morning. Their experiences of positive emotions increased, and their overall life satisfaction improved.

---

On the other hand, eudaimonic wellbeing emphasises living a life of virtue and purpose, often linked to concepts, such as self-actualisation and personal growth. A prominent eudaimonic model is the Psychological Wellbeing model (Ryff, 1995), which explores what makes life worth living in contrast to the transient nature of emotions, upon which the Subjective Wellbeing model is based (Diener, 2018). This comprehensive model consists of six elements:

autonomy, personal growth, environmental mastery, purpose in life, positive relationships, and self-acceptance. Drawing from extensive literature reviews and theories from such prominent psychologists and psychotherapists as Adler, Freud, and Maslow, it provides a perspective on wellbeing that goes beyond simple happiness.

Emerging research suggests a link between some lifestyle medicine pillars and psychological wellbeing, with some authors suggesting that it's not the diet but mental health that can help some individuals maintain healthy weight (Rand et al., 2017). A systematic review of positive psychological concepts assessed among almost 60 thousand participants showed that improvements in wellbeing were associated with lifestyle changes (Conradson et al., 2022). For example, research with obese patients exploring the impact of psychological wellbeing on their obesity showed that autonomy played an essential role in maintaining a weight-loss programme (Zhu et al., 2022). The deficit in autonomy meant that individuals felt excessively dependable on others to help them with weight loss resulting in their journey of weight loss being hindered. At the same time, when patients developed too much autonomy, the belief that they could do it by themselves, this often stopped them from continuing to attend a weight-loss programme. The study suggested that interventions aiming to support weight loss should also address individuals' psychological needs and help them strike a balance in their autonomy.

Similar findings were observed regarding substance use. Adolescents who engaged in excessive drinking often reported a decline in many aspects of wellbeing, such as life purpose; at the same time, they also reported having particularly close relationships with others (Gostoli et al., 2021). Their lively social network increased their susceptibility to peer pressure, making them more likely to engage in substance use. Subsequently, researchers designed a combined programme comprising wellbeing and lifestyle interventions to reduce substance use in young people (Fantini et al., 2024). Participants were divided into three groups: one without any intervention, the second one receiving a lifestyle intervention only, and the third one receiving a wellbeing therapy intervention only. Both the lifestyle and wellbeing interventions led to lower odds of binge drinking after six months. Notably, only the wellbeing therapy intervention provided a protective effect against cannabis use post-intervention.

This finding highlights the crucial role of wellbeing in preventing substance abuse. However, further studies are needed to explore the intricacies of this approach.

### Liam's journey

*Liam, a 15-year-old boy living in a small Irish town, struggled with self-doubt and insecurity most of his life. Though he found solace in the beautiful Irish nature and enjoyed walks and connecting with his surroundings, he felt like an outsider among people, and especially at school. His struggle with self-acceptance began early, watching his friends navigate life with ease while he grappled with self-doubt and loneliness. This pressure led him to try e-cigarettes, with a hope of earning his friends' acceptance. While, initially, they made him feel better, soon he became addicted to them.*

*Liam knew it was not good for him so he confided in his mother and asked her for help. She signed him up to the wellbeing group therapy, which focused his attention on developing positive relationships, life purpose, and overall wellbeing. In this supportive environment, he began to understand what it meant to be accepting and compassionate towards himself and value the unique person he had become.*

*Over months, Liam's urge to use e-cigarettes diminished as he found healthier ways to cope with stress. The therapy sessions bolstered his self-worth and clarity about his future. He rediscovered joy in playing his guitar, exploring the countryside and spending time with friends who valued him, unlike those who brought out the worst in him.*

*The impact of wellbeing therapy extended beyond personal growth. Liam's family relationships improved; he reconnected with his passion for learning and became more involved in school activities, finding new interests and hobbies that enriched his life.*

With the advancement of positive psychology, there is a growing recognition of the need to integrate both hedonic and eudaimonic dimensions of wellbeing. Martin Seligman's original Authentic Happiness model (2002) initially aimed at helping people increase happiness levels by living a life of pleasure, purpose, and meaning. However, a decade later, influenced by advancements in psychology, Seligman acknowledged that happiness alone is insufficient, advocating for a focus on flourishing instead. This shift led to the development of the Wellbeing Model (Seligman, 2011), which emphasises enabling individuals to flourish rather than merely seeking happiness. The model posits that true wellbeing, or "the good life", entails flourishing, which is the highest state of wellbeing combing both psychological and emotional dimensions. The Wellbeing Model comprises five key elements: positive emotions, engagement, relationships, meaning, and accomplishment. Flourishing, according to Seligman, is also intrinsically motivating to individuals, meaning that the pursuit of flourishing is an enjoyable and sought-after journey for them.

While Seligman's model is most popular in positive psychology, other models of flourishing include Keyes' Mental Health Continuum (2002), as detailed in Chapter 1, and Diener et al.'s Flourishing Scale (2009), which incorporates elements such as purpose and meaning, social relationships, contribution to others, positive self-image, and optimism. Additionally, another model, tested with tens of thousands of participants, defined flourishing as consisting of essential elements such as positive emotions, engagement, interest, meaning, and purpose, along with additional features like self-esteem, optimism, resilience, vitality, self-determination, and positive relationships (Huppert & So, 2013). These models collectively explore diverse aspects of wellbeing, with some overlapping components and others presenting nuanced perspectives.

---

### BEST POSSIBLE HEALTH

#### (Adapted from Gibson et al., 2021)

Begin by deeply reflecting on your current health status. Envision your best possible self, picturing a version of you in excellent health, haven taken exceptional care of your body. You exercise regularly and maintain a balanced diet. Through dedication and effort, you have achieved all your health-related goals. Reflect on the sense of accomplishment and the positive feelings of being fit and healthy. Now, consider the essential steps you took to reach this point.

Please spend the next 10 minutes writing continuously about what you imagined, using the following tips to guide you:

1. Be as creative and imaginative as you wish. Don't worry about perfect grammar or spelling; this exercise is for personal use. Sharing and discussing your ideas with trusted friends, family, or your healthcare team is beneficial.

2. Feel free to write everything down on your first attempt. As you repeat this exercise, more ideas will naturally come to you.

3. Remember, the path to success is often paved with small steps. It might be easier to start with achievable goals, such as investing in a pedometer or trying new, healthier recipes more often. However, if you want to set ambitious goals, like running a half-marathon, that's perfectly fine, too. The key is setting clear, achievable goals to guide your health journey. If one aspect of your health feels challenging, focus on another. The key is to write about long-term goals to make noticeable improvements over time.

In a recent study, Oishi and Westgate (2022) introduced an alternative perspective on wellbeing, highlighting the significance of psychological richness – moments of paradigm shifts, those 'aha' moments that elevate wellbeing beyond traditional eudaimonic and hedonic factors. Emerging research indicates a correlation between certain aspects of lifestyle medicine and psychological richness. For instance, amidst the COVID-19 pandemic, experiencing psychological richness helped shield individuals from stress and the inclination to withdraw from social contact (Gu et al., 2023). Furthermore, those who incorporated psychological richness into their lives were more likely to recover from COVID-19 (Dahlen & Thorbjørnsen, 2022). Thus, psychological richness offers an alternative to the dichotomous models of flourishing and can also potentially add to the science of positive health.

While wellbeing models offer valuable insights, they have significant limitations. They depend on componential frameworks, leading to discrepancies across models. Also, these models frequently assume a universal intrinsic motivation for wellbeing, which may only apply in some contexts. Additionally, they overlook the complexity of human nature and the impact of wellbeing models within other psychological theories. Currently, the highest levels of wellbeing are considered more beneficial than moderate levels, disregarding the importance of moderation. Finally, they do not consider the benefits of adverse states, which limits their perspective on the human psyche. Overall, these challenges can result in a flawed understanding of flourishing, as such these limitations need to be considered when applying flourishing models in the context of positive health.

Despite their limitations, it's important to note these models can still provide a good foundation for understanding wellbeing. They serve as a groundwork for exploring the interaction between lifestyle medicine and positive psychology in promoting positive health of individuals who are healthy and those experiencing various health conditions. In this chapter we will explore some of the elements of these models that are important to positive health and ways in which we can combine positive psychology and lifestyle medicine to create positive mental health.

## CORE ELEMENTS OF FLOURISHING IN POSITIVE HEALTH

### POSITIVE EMOTIONS

With the rise in research focusing on the positive aspects of well-being, there has been an increased recognition of a wide range of positive emotions and the role they play in daily life and our health. One of the most prominent theories of emotions, explored in the context of facial expressions, was proposed by Ekman (1992) who identified six basic emotions: anger, surprise, disgust, enjoyment, fear, and sadness. Most of these emotions were negative, and a significant body of research delved deeper into them. The primary driver for this research was the evolutionary reasons for negative emotions that helped individuals and generations to survive. Positive emotions, on the other hand, were seen in a simplistic way as just keeping us happy.

However, amidst the avalanche of research focused on the benefits of negative emotions emerged a series of studies by Isen (1999), which focused on the benefits of positive emotions beyond simplistic happiness. Then, following Isen's lead, the Broaden-and-Build theory was developed (Fredrickson, 2001), which has explored three fundamental benefits of positive emotions.

## BROADEN-AND-BUILD THEORY

The Broaden-and-Build Theory of Positive Emotions (Fredrickson, 2001) posits that positive emotions such as joy, interest, and love expand an individual's momentary thought–action repertoire. This means that when people experience positive emotions, their thinking becomes more creative, flexible, and they are more open to new possibilities. This broadened perspective allows individuals to explore their environment, engage in novel activities, and build stronger connections with others. Unlike negative emotions, which narrow focus to specific survival actions, positive emotions encourage exploratory behaviours and innovative thinking.

The second benefit of positive emotions is their "undoing" effect, according to which positive emotions can help mitigate or "undo" the physiological impact of negative emotions. For example, when individuals experience stress or negative emotions, their bodies exhibit heightened physiological responses such as increased heart rate and muscle tension. Positive emotions, such as joy or contentment, can quickly reduce these stress responses, helping the body return to a more relaxed state. This effect alleviates immediate stress and contributes to overall health and wellbeing by promoting faster recovery from adverse emotional states.

Thirdly, over time, the broadened mindset fostered by the experiences of positive emotions helps individuals build lasting personal resources, including physical health, intellectual abilities, social bonds, and psychological resilience. For example, research showed that positive emotions protect us against colds (Cohen et al., 2003). In an experiment with students, half of them were injected with a common flu virus. Those who experienced more positive emotions at the onset of the experiment have also reported milder symptoms of illness and faster recovery. These accumulative resources enhance overall wellbeing and provide a buffer against future adversities. Essentially, positive emotions not only improve immediate mood but also contribute to long-term personal growth and resilience, creating an upward spiral of positivity.

---

### RECALL ACTS OF KINDNESS

#### (Adapted from Ko et al., 2019)

Over the next three days, set aside a few moments to reminisce about a past act of kindness you offered someone. Delve deeply into this memory, paying close attention to the thoughts and emotions you experienced during that moment. This simple activity will help you re-experience these positive emotions and will help you benefit from your acts of kindness over and over again.

---

Following the Broaden-and-Build theory, further research was conducted that aimed to expand our understanding of positive emotions. For example, Fredrickson and Losada (2005) proposed a nonlinear model showing that flourishing individuals experienced a ratio of 2.9 positive emotions to every negative emotion. In contrast, those not flourishing fell below this ratio during a 28-day assessment. This model faced significant criticism, particularly regarding the equation used to determine the 3:1 ratio (Brown et al., 2013). Despite the debate over exact figures, the core idea exists and Fredrickson (2001) warned not to throw a baby out with the bath water. Studies over many decades identified a similar ratio, e.g. the Gottman love lab (Gottman, 2000) researching happy couples provided a 5:1 ratio predicting lasting marriages. Even if we put the ratio debate aside, individuals who experience higher levels of negative emotions compared to positive tend to report poor mental health. This principle is supported by research on subjective wellbeing showing that the balance between positive and negative emotions is more important than the experiences of these emotions (Diener et al., 2018). For instance, a person enduring chronic pain may still flourish psychologically as their life is filled with an abundance of positive emotions they experience through activities like connecting with their loved ones, engaging with nature, or maintaining a positive outlook, even though their pain persists. Thus, it is the balance of positive emotions that matters and that could contribute significantly to developing positive health. For more evidence of the impact of positive emotions on health, please explore the research reviewed by Sarah Pressman et al. (2019).

## EMOTIONAL NUANCES

Understanding emotions goes beyond experiencing them; it involves recognising the emotions, labelling them and then managing them effectively. Emotional granularity highlights this ability, as it is akin to having a finely tuned emotional radar. For instance, individuals with high emotional granularity can differentiate between feeling angry, afraid, tired, or lonely. In contrast, those with lower granularity might generalise these negative emotions under the broad label of "feeling bad".

Emotional granularity and emotion labelling also represent different components of emotional intelligence. Emotion labelling is the ability to recognise and name specific emotional states. Those skilled in this can accurately identify their feelings as anger, joy, sadness, or fear. This skill is a foundation for developing emotional intelligence and enhancing interpersonal communication. In fact, recent research indicates that the extent of emotional words an individual uses is associated with higher levels of mental health (Ikeda, 2023). By precisely expressing their emotional states, individuals can, therefore, better convey their feelings to others, fostering understanding and empathy in their relationships. This skill can also help individuals with a process of self-acceptance.

On the other hand, emotional granularity is more than just categorising emotions – it is about understanding the nuanced gradations and subtleties within them. This advanced skill involves recognising and labelling primary emotional states and discerning finer distinctions. For example, people with high emotional granularity can differentiate between feelings of frustration, irritation, or disappointment, while those with limited emotional granularity might group these nuanced emotions under broader labels like "anger" or "upset". This level of understanding not only empowers individuals to navigate their emotional landscape with precision and control, but also instils a sense of capability and self-assurance.

While emotion labelling fosters emotional literacy and communication, emotional granularity elevates this ability by enabling individuals to navigate the intricacies of their emotional life experiences.

---

**Daily boosts**: In a study examining the daily experiences of individuals who flourished psychologically versus those who did not, researchers discovered significant differences. Flourishing individuals exhibited more daily "boosts" in positive emotions in response to everyday pleasant events such as acts of kindness, social interactions, leisure activities, learning, or spiritual engagement. In other words, they reacted with more 'oomph' to their daily experiences. These findings imply that enhancing wellbeing may be influenced by subtle yet meaningful changes in our emotional responses to everyday moments of positivity. For more information, go to Catalino and Fredrickson (2011).

---

Research suggests that emotional granularity is associated with numerous psychological benefits. For example, individuals with higher emotional granularity tend to experience better emotional regulation, have stronger social relationships, and exhibit fewer symptoms of depression and anxiety (Kashdan et al., 2015). This ability to identify and articulate emotions accurately can lead to more effective problem-solving and coping strategies in stressful situations. Consider fear, for example. When faced with an aggressive dog barking at you, feeling fearful might prompt you to flee immediately. However, fleeing would not be beneficial in a different scenario, such as feeling fearful before undergoing surgery. The ability to adapt our responses according to the situation is important for our survival and personal development. For instance, recognising heightened arousal as a signal to act swiftly during emergencies or as an indication that we should remain composed and focused is essential (Jamieson et al., 2018). This nuanced comprehension of emotions empowers us to make appropriate decisions.

Furthermore, this emotional granularity is also linked to improved levels of respiratory sinus arrhythmia, better known as the vagal tone, which is also responsible for our overall mental and physical health (Hoemann et al., 2021). People with higher levels of emotional granularity are more tuned to their bodies. They show a greater variety of ways in which they behave when sitting or resting, thus allowing them to use the most appropriate strategy in each situation that requires relaxation. Moreover, it is as if they have a fine-tuned radar that helps them discern as to what is happening inside them. The more finely tuned they are, the more different kinds of heart and breathing patterns they experience when sitting down, and the better they were at recognising how their bodies feel.

In addition to the theoretical research, a variety of interventions have been designed that aimed at enhancing individuals' positive wellbeing. Many of these interventions focus on acknowledging or labelling emotions. For example, the "counting your blessings" intervention (Emmons & McCullough, 2003) demonstrated that expressing gratitude improved positive health outcomes compared to individuals who dwell on daily stresses instead. Similarly, activities associated with participants practising expressive writing result in more significant emotional disclosure, which in turn helps them cope more effectively with daily stress (Pennebaker & Francis, 1996). Furthermore, research indicates significant health advantages of focusing on the positive aspects of traumatic events. Those who reflect on it, visited medical professionals less frequently for three months after the experiment (King & Miner, 2000). Moreover, caregivers who articulated their experiences with more positive emotions following the loss of their partners to AIDS showed higher morale and a reduced likelihood of depression (Stein et al., 1997). Therefore, existing research emphasises the importance of these experiences and the expression of positive emotions in fostering overall health and wellbeing.

### OPTIMISM

Imagine a world where the way we interpret events could shape our health. This is the power of explanatory style, a concept we delve into in this chapter. It is not just a narrative we construct about the reasons behind events but a lens through which we view the world. This concept, born from the theory of learned helplessness (Seligman, 1975), has evolved into a tool for optimistic thinking (Seligman, 1998). Let us explore its three fundamental components:

1. **Internal vs. External**: This facet relates to whether we attribute the cause of an event to factors within ourselves (internal) or external circumstances. Consider this scenario: When someone struggles with sleeping, they might ascribe it to external factors like noise or excessive light in their bedroom or internal factors such as insomnia (reflecting a pessimistic thinking style). Identifying as an insomniac suggests a shift in self-perception, indicating a perceived lack of control over their situation, which could hinder their efforts to initiate changes.

2. **Stable vs. Unstable**: This dimension explores whether we view the cause of a situation as permanent (stable) or subject to change (unstable). For instance, if faced with failure to moderate alcohol, perceiving oneself as inherently lacking the ability to stop drinking reflects a stable explanation, whereas acknowledging that it was just a choice we made on the night suggests an unstable perspective.

3. **Global vs. Specific**: This aspect of explanatory styles delves into whether we believe the cause of an event has ramifications across all aspects of our lives (global) or is confined to a particular situation (specific). For instance, spilling coffee and interpreting it as a sign of perpetual clumsiness represents a global explanation of the negative situation, whereas viewing it as a one-off incident shows that we are able to compartmentalise our failures and recognise that it is just one aspect of our lives that is affected.

Combining these elements indicates our optimism or pessimism. In some cases, we may be optimistic in one element and pessimistic in another. For example, we may believe that bad times last forever (pessimistic) but we also are able to attribute negative outcomes to specific aspects of our lives (optimistic). We could also be optimistic in one situation but pessimistic in another. For example, we may have tried to lose weight for years without success. Therefore, we tend to believe that successful weight loss is beyond our reach, reflecting a pessimistic outlook. However, we approach challenges at work with optimism, as these are not burdened by the emotional complexities tied to weight loss. This is why examining these explanatory styles in the context of positive health is crucial, as the factors influencing lifestyle habits may stem from the psychological constraints of pessimistic thinking.

Optimistic thinking style impacts not only our mind, but also our body. Pessimistic explanatory style negatively influences Immunoglobulin A (IgA), a crucial antibody for maintaining health (Brennan & Charnetski, 2000). This means that continuously assigning blame to oneself for adverse events and perceiving them as enduring stressors significantly undermines the production of antibodies like IgA, increasing susceptibility to illnesses. Furthermore, pessimistic thinking influences cell-mediated immunity (CMI), another critical immune system component (Kamen-Siegel et al., 1991). Similar to the findings regarding IgA, consistently attributing adverse events to oneself and experiencing prolonged distress associated with it, can disrupt immune function, impairing the body's ability to combat infections and diseases. As such, optimistic thinking can help our bodies deal more effectively with infections. Therefore, it is not solely about the events themselves, or the lifestyle we live, but also about our cognitive interpretations of the events or our lifestyle, which significantly influence our chances of maintaining optimal positive health.

---

**Coronary artery bypass**: Patients undergoing coronary artery bypass surgery were evaluated one day before the procedure, 6 to 8 days post-operation, and again six months later. Optimistic thinking in these patients predicted more problem-focused coping, a faster physical recovery, and a quicker return to normal life activities after discharge. For more information, refer to Scheier et al., 1989.

---

## FLOW

At the core of positive health lies the concept of "flow". Psychological flow is a state of mind where an individual is fully absorbed, focused, and engaged in an activity, deriving immense pleasure from it. Interestingly, this enjoyment is often realised after the activity as, during it, they are so engrossed in the task that they are oblivious to it. This state, commonly referred to as "being in the zone", entails a complete immersion where their minds are not wandering, external distractions tend to fade away, and they experience a deep sense of control and satisfaction.

The rewards of flow are not just limited to the activity itself, but extend towards higher levels of pleasure, enhanced intrinsic motivation, and improved performance. This is particularly relevant in the context of positive health. The more enjoyment and intrinsic motivation individuals find in lifestyle changes, the more likely they are to maintain them, leading to a healthier and more fulfilling life.

Consider someone who wants to increase their level of physical activity. According to flow theory, it's crucial for them to match their skill level to the activity they choose. If their skill level is too high for the activity, they will become bored and lose interest. Conversely, if they lack the necessary skills for the activity, they will feel anxious, which can either discourage them from continuing or lead to mental health issues. However, the ideal state, known as "flow", occurs when their skills are perfectly matched to the challenge of the activity. In this state, they become fully immersed, enjoy the process, and continually improve their skills while maintaining healthy behaviour. This shows that flow can be a powerful tool in overcoming challenges and achieving personal growth.

The connection between physical activity and flow is not one-sided. Engaging in higher levels of physical activity increases the likelihood of experiencing flow, particularly among athletes and inactive individuals (Elbe et al., 2010). Athletes, for instance, often adopt a task-oriented approach and set clear goals for improvement, which fosters the experience of flow (Stavrou et al., 2015). Similarly, individuals who partake in recreational physical activities frequently encounter more flow-like episodes and find these experiences enjoyable. This also applies to inactive individuals who participate in individual or team sports (Decloe et al., 2009; Elbe et al., 2010). These findings suggest that physical activity not only promotes flow experiences but also helps individuals sustain their new behaviours through intrinsic motivation. Hence, flow is a crucial element in not just enhancing lifestyle but also improving positive health outcomes.

### HARMONIOUS PASSION AND FLOW

Passion is "a strong inclination towards an activity people like, find important, and invest time and energy" (Vallerand et al., 2003, p. 757). Passion is harmonious when the activity is under the control of the individual. In contrast, passion is obsessive when the activity controls the individual (Fernet et al., 2014). This dualistic model of passion (Vallerand et al., 2003) conceptualises it as either obsessive or harmonious based on the individual's sense of control over their passion. These distinctions result in different outcomes. Those with obsessive passion tend to reduce their experiences of positive emotions associated with their interest and success associated with accomplishing something related to their passion. In contrast, those with harmonious passion savour these moments boosting their positive emotions (Schellenberg et al., 2020).

Obsessive passion often leads to negative emotions, such as guilt about not engaging in the activity or shame if performance falls short of expectations. This type of passion can be a double-edged sword, leading to accomplishments and achievements (Li, 2010), but also potentially reducing wellbeing. In contrast, harmonious passion is linked to positive emotions, as individuals are better able to manage their urges and maintain a balanced approach to their passion, thereby enhancing wellbeing (Vallerand et al., 2007).

In positive health, fostering harmonious passion is not just beneficial, it's empowering. It not only promotes better mental health and emotional wellbeing but also supports sustained engagement and enjoyment in activities, which is particularly beneficial when individuals strive to change their lifestyle behaviour. By maintaining control over their passion and balancing it with other aspects of life, individuals can achieve a healthier and more fulfilling lifestyle, taking charge of their wellbeing.

Flow, a state of complete absorption and enjoyment in an activity, is primarily associated with harmonious passion (Carpentier et al., 2012). While both obsessively and harmoniously passionate individuals can experience flow, those with obsessive passion typically only achieve it in the activity they are fixated on. In contrast, harmoniously passionate individuals are able to experience flow across various aspects of their lives. This ability to achieve flow in multiple areas significantly contributes to their overall wellbeing, highlighting the positive impact of harmonious passion on individuals' health and happiness. This further emphasises the benefits of fostering a harmonious passion for a more fulfilling healthy lifestyle.

## POSITIVE RELATIONSHIPS

Christopher Peterson, a pioneer in positive psychology, is renowned for his motto, "Other people matter", which highlights the transformative power of connection and meaningful relationships which facilitates wellbeing (Peterson, 2013). Our intrinsic need for connection not only helps us form meaningful interpersonal bonds but also has the potential to significantly improve our health (Ryan & Deci, 2000). The satisfaction or frustration of this need profoundly shapes our life experiences and health outcomes. When fulfilled, we experience a sense of belonging, whereas its absence leaves us feeling isolated and excluded (Schmidt & Häggström, 2022). Consequently, interventions targeting relationships must address the needs of both groups. Those grappling with frustration of connecting may require cognitive restructuring to overcome self-limiting beliefs about connecting with others and developing friendships, while those satisfied with their relationships can benefit from strategies to sustain positivity and thrive in their relationships.

Irrespective of personality, the presence of others contributes to an increase in happiness, with peak happiness often occurring during social interactions (Kahneman & Riis, 2005). Community setting are particularly beneficial as they enhance joy by amplifying laughter and social connections (Provine, 2000). Furthermore, relationships provide invaluable support, with the need for it decreasing with age (Keyes, 2002). Longitudinal studies point to the lasting influence of supportive relationships, whether nurtured in childhood or discovered in adulthood, in promoting personal growth and resilience (Werner, 1993; Vaillant & Mukamal, 2003). Therefore, connecting with others and nurturing relationships is crucial to our wellbeing.

---

### GIFT OF TIME

#### (Gander et al., 2013)

During the upcoming week, prioritise spending quality time with three individuals who are important to you – whether they're friends, family members, or colleagues. Ensure that these interactions are additional to your existing plans, allowing you to genuinely devote yourself to connecting with them.

---

Apart from improving overall wellbeing, evidence indicates that happiness is also contagious, thus when we connect with others, we can influence how happy they will feel. A longitudinal study spanning two decades, involving nearly 5,000 individuals, revealed that the happiness of one person within a social network can significantly impact the happiness of others within the network, even without direct interaction (Fowler & Christakis, 2009). This ripple effect extends up to three degrees of separation. Specifically, when a person's immediate friends experience increased happiness, it correlates with a 15% rise in the individual's own happiness. Similarly, when the friends of those friends become happier, it results in a 10% increase in the individual's happiness. Moreover, the study found that the happiness of individuals within close proximity has the most substantial impact on us. For instance, if your friend who resides within a mile radius becomes happier, it increases your likelihood of becoming happier by 25%. Furthermore, the happiness of next-door neighbours seems to have an even greater effect, boosting our wellbeing by 34%. Therefore, the interconnected nature of human happiness means that the people we spend time with have a profound influence on our emotional states, happiness, and perhaps even positive health, highlighting the significance of the quality of our relationships.

**Adam's story**

*Adam lived in Minnesota (USA). He was a man of ambition and dreams, and he led a healthy life apart from one habit: smoking.*

*From the moment Adam woke to the time he fell sleep, the craving for nicotine gnawed at him. It was not just a physical need, but a psychological dependence associated with his daily habits and social interactions.*

*Adam's friends who were his closest companions were all smokers. Every gathering, every celebration, and every moment of his past time was associated with cigarettes and the fun they all had blowing circles of smoke.*

*He tried to quit. Each attempt was a battle against himself, against the years of conditioning. However, every time he mustered the strength to resist, his friends' habits dragged him back into the cycle of addiction.*

*With each failed attempt, Adam's spirit grew heavier, burdened by his shortcomings. He felt like a prisoner in his own body, longing for freedom but unable to break free from this habit.*

## THE NUANCES OF CONNECTION

Social prescribing initiatives – prescribing a range of non-clinical community supports or activities which can have significant health and wellbeing effects – are introduced by governments globally, aiming to improve health and wellbeing while tackling health inequalities and potentially reducing long-term healthcare expenses. While it seems intuitive that encouraging social connections could enhance wellbeing, evidence for social prescribing is mixed.

A comprehensive review by Kiely et al. (2022) explored medical studies, websites, and reports on social prescribing projects. Surprisingly, half of the studies that were examined in this review failed to demonstrate positive health impacts. Particularly concerning was the lack of improvement in mental health outcomes across most studies that explored social prescribing. These findings highlighted a crucial context to social prescribing: merely connecting with people and having them in our lives does not guarantee better health and wellbeing.

For instance, recent research on positivity resonance indicates that brief interactions, even with strangers, can increase wellbeing on a physiological level (Major et al., 2018). However, the exchange of moments of positivity within these interactions is pivotal. Conversely, relationships filled with criticism, conflict, or excessive demands can induce detrimental stress that outweighs connection benefits (Lincoln et al., 2003). Thus, the critical factor lies not in mere connection or the presence of people in one's life but in the quality of social support and interactions between individuals, which profoundly impact positive health outcomes.

**IMPROVING CONNECTIONS**

Active-Constructive Responding is one of the most popular interventions that aims to enhance the quality of our interpersonal connections (Gable et al., 2004). This model highlights four distinct ways we typically react to the good news shared by our loved ones, friends, or colleagues:

1. The passive-destructive response deflects the topic, scarcely acknowledging the shared good news.
2. The passive-constructive response is characterised by a nonchalant acknowledgement without much ado.
3. The active-destructive reaction involves dampening the mood by highlighting potential drawbacks of the good news.
4. The active-constructive response is about an enthusiastic and engaged reaction to the good news, fostering connection and positivity.

Studies show that only the fourth approach, the active-constructive response, fosters flourishing relationships. All other approaches diminish positivity in human interaction. Therefore, to re-connect with people who matter and improve your relationships with others, it is useful to start practising this approach, even if it feels unnatural at first.

Within the framework of positive health, this approach is crucial as it reminds us to reflect not only on whether we have people in our social network but also how much support we receive from them. Consider an individual seeking to adopt stress management techniques, only to face ridicule or indifference from their social circle. Depending on their disposition, they might persevere or withdraw from such endeavours straight away. Hence, fostering an integrated approach to lifestyle modifications, including social support, is crucial when aiming to enhance positive health outcomes.

In positive health, social support is needed to encourage lifestyle changes. Thus, positive health interventions could centre on developing and nurturing positive relationships via practising kindness. Beyond the relational benefits, engaging in acts of kindness profoundly impacts individuals' overall wellbeing. While conventional wisdom may suggest self-indulgence during distress (e.g. having a treat, or going shopping to relieve stress), empirical evidence refutes this notion (Nelson et al., 2016). Instead, redirecting our attention outward by embracing altruistic actions, and integrating acts of kindness into our daily lives can be a powerful tool for changing lifestyles and bringing more positive health into our lives. Such practices can also significantly elevate wellbeing.

Various suggestions exist for incorporating acts of kindness into our daily routines, ranging from purchasing a meal for a homeless individual to donating goods, engaging in social recycling, or participating in random acts of kindness (Curry et al., 2018). Interestingly, the effectiveness of these acts is magnified when we perform 3–5 acts of kindness on one day rather than disperse them over a week (Lyubomirsky et al., 2005). Thus, in the context of positive health and the support necessary for lifestyle changes, embracing acts of kindness is a powerful tool for fostering wellbeing and nurturing supportive relationships. Ultimately, it is not merely about the presence of others in our lives but rather about cultivating relationships that offer meaningful support.

## MEANING AND PURPOSE IN LIFE

What is the meaning of life? To some, it signifies fulfilling personal aspirations and cherished goals (Ryff & Singer, 1998). Others perceive it as discovering the inherent order and significance woven into our existence (Reker & Wong, 1988). Another perspective views it as a life imbued with purpose, significance, and coherence

(Heintzelman & King, 2014). Regardless of the definition, meaning in life is a crucial aspect of a positive health journey.

The predominant understanding of the meaning of life centres around experiencing self-awareness of how aspects of our lives impact each other and having a clear life purpose (Steger et al., 2015). This entails gaining insight into our identity, understanding our reason for being, identifying our core values that could relate to our health, mapping out our positive health and other life aspirations, and acknowledging how our life experiences have shaped us into becoming our current selves. While meaning delves into our existence's philosophical and existential aspects of life, purpose is about the application of meaning in our daily lives, which can impact our overall wellbeing.

Moreover, it is crucial to differentiate between the meaning in life and the meaning of life itself. Meaning in life refers to what is important in our life experience experiences, while meaning of life grapples with existential questions about the nature of our existence. Thus, in good health, we focus our discussions on the meaning in life.

Realising the meaning in our lives strongly correlates with elevated levels of physical wellbeing (Roepke et al., 2014). It serves as a buffer against various pathologies and enhances multiple dimensions of our overall wellbeing (Steger, 2017). Additionally, a reciprocal relationship exists between a good mood and a deepened sense of meaning in life (Hicks & King, 2009). Thus, having a meaning is not only an eudaimonic process but also contributes to hedonic wellness and health.

---

### MOST FEARED OBITUARY
#### (Adapted from Frisch, 2005)

Think of a scenario where you have yet to succeed in changing your unhealthy and unhappy behavioural patterns before your death. Reflect on your current habits and routines that contribute to your discontent, and visualise the consequences of these issues going forward. Picture a long life where you persist in living without making any positive adjustments. Your standards, priorities, and goals remain unchanged while your happiness and health steadily decline.

Now, write your own obituary with all the intricate detail. Consider that your family, friends, and strangers will read it in newspapers and online. Write about your life as it would unfold if you continued living in the same unhealthy and unhappy way without any changes.

Crucially, during challenging times, meaning provides significant protection for our mental health (Wong, 2011), surpassing even the impact of experiencing positive emotions or other elements of wellbeing. It enables us to find purpose and coherence amid suffering, which in turn supports our psychological resilience.

It is important to note, however, that while the presence of life meaning is linked to higher levels of wellbeing, actively searching for meaning can have the opposite effect (Li et al., 2021). Thus, in the process of improving positive health or changing lifestyle, an exploration of meaning in life could have a temporary negative impact on individuals. It is also important to consider that discussing the concept of meaning could benefit those who are clear about their meaning in life or their purpose but have not yet connected it with their positive health goals.

Life purpose is a practical and motivational dimension of finding meaning in life (Steger, 2012). Purpose is intimately linked with the goals we set for ourselves. Without a clear sense of purpose, even if we have a broader meaning in life, we may lack the resolve or fortitude to pursue what truly matters to us. This is where the life purpose comes in. Conversely, if we have a defined life purpose but lack a sense of meaning behind it, we might eventually realise our actions and values are incongruent. Therefore, it is crucial to consider not only what matters in our lives and what our intentions for a good life are, but also how fulfilling our journey of achieving them is.

The optimal scenario is about aligning our meaning and purpose simultaneously. This alignment empowers us to live with clarity of our meaning and fulfilment as we pursue goals that resonate deeply with our sense of purpose and overarching meaning in life, which can support our efforts of improving our positive health.

## THE "HOW" OF FLOURISHING

### COMBINING POSITIVE PSYCHOLOGY AND LIFESTYLE MEDICINE TO CREATE POSITIVE MENTAL HEALTH

Positive health sciences are currently in their infancy. We draw from two well-established disciplines with substantial research and practice. Positive psychology has been evolving for nearly three decades which resulted in publishing tens of thousands of scientific articles. Similarly, lifestyle medicine has expanded rapidly, becoming the fastest-growing speciality in medicine, and is grounded in decades of research across six distinct areas of medicine akin to their pillars. Both fields have extensively explored various topics, demonstrating their impact on wellbeing and health respectively. However, more research is needed that integrates these two fields into a cohesive approach, which is the essence of positive health.

Various lifestyle medicine specialists have advocated integrating positive psychology with lifestyle medicine (e.g., Lianov et al., 2019; Morton, 2018). They highlighted the parallels between the fields and encouraged researchers and practitioners to combine their approaches. This integration is particularly significant because both fields have developed several interventions, and the potential health and wellbeing benefits that could be achieved through their application together are substantial.

The first evidence of combining positive psychology and lifestyle medicine interventions came from Przybylko and colleagues (2020), who developed a ten-week programme alternating between interventions from both fields. Participants engaged in daily and weekly challenges. During positive psychology weeks, they practised, such interventions as gratitude and connection with nature or performing acts of kindness. During lifestyle medicine weeks, they exercised moderately, aiming for 10,000 steps, ate eight servings of plant-based food, or relaxed in quiet places. Results showed that the intervention group experienced a 17.2% increase in flourishing compared to the control group. Additionally, at a 12-week follow-up, participants maintained their increased flourishing levels while the control group's levels declined. This study was the first to demonstrate that a combined positive psychology and lifestyle medicine intervention can enhance flourishing and improve diet and physical activity.

Building on these findings, our RCSI Centre for positive health Sciences conducted a pilot study with adolescents (Burke & Dunne, 2024), building on the approach of modifying existing lifestyle medicine interventions to incorporate elements of positive psychology. For instance, we encouraged participants to perform acts of kindness toward their bodies and reflect on how to include psychobiotics in their meals, instead of simply advocating for a healthy diet with psychobiotics. Our results demonstrated that overall wellbeing improved in participants who engaged in a combination of activities, compared to those practising only lifestyle medicine interventions or those in the wait-control group. However, participants' satisfaction with the pillars of lifestyle medicine, e.g. eating well or sleeping well, either declined or remained unchanged after the four-week programme. As such, the study showed that looking after our mind and body does not necessarily result in similar outcomes. These results also indicate that positive psychology and lifestyle medicine may operate through different mechanisms. While combining both might seem beneficial, the mixture could improve or diminish their health and wellbeing impacts.

Additionally, more research is needed to explore the impact of well-known positive psychology interventions on lifestyle medicine outcomes, such as good sleep, eating well or substance use. Furthermore, establishing pathways for practising positive health in an integrated way is essential. In the meantime, we can use existing models from both fields and investigate how they can be used to improve health and wellbeing. The remainder of this chapter will explore these possibilities.

## POSITIVE EMOTION REGULATION

If you've ever been in nature but couldn't connect with its beauty because you were overwhelmed by persistent, upsetting thoughts, or flooded with negative emotions, you're not alone. Many of us have experienced this, and it's a sign that we're missing out on daily opportunities to enhance our wellbeing. The good news is that we have the power to change this. By putting in a little more effort, we can truly maximise these moments. This is the same principle upon which a five-step process for practising positive interventions (Quoidbach et al., 2015) is based. It assumes that positive experiences are not enough to improve our wellbeing, as we need to engage additional processes to optimise their impact. Let's explore it in more detail.

**Situation selection** involves choosing daily activities that foster positive outcomes for you. For example, this could mean spending a quiet evening with a loved one, attending an event you enjoy like a comedy show, or engaging in activities supporting a healthy lifestyle, such as running or planning a plant-based menu for the family for a week.

**Situation modification** involves adjusting an experience to maximise its benefits for wellbeing. For instance, if you're attending a comedy gig, to modify this situation and optimise its impact, you can choose a comedian you know and enjoy. If you're going for a run, opt for a local park instead of a treadmill. When preparing a plant-based menu, review your favourite recipe books and find recipes with all the fruits and vegetables you enjoy most.

**Attentional deployment** involves paying particular attention to the moment and being mindful rather than mindless when engaging in a positive activity. At a comedy gig, this means pausing occasionally to absorb the experience with all your senses fully. When running, it's about focusing on your body and how it moves or noticing the beauty of your surroundings. While preparing food or a menu, it's about being fully present in the moment and taking your time when exploring each recipe.

**Cognitive change** involves reframing a situation to maximise its positivity. This could mean feeling grateful for the opportunity to engage in an activity, appreciating how it allows your character strengths to shine, or recognising the emotions you experience, such as awe while running in a park or acknowledging a burst of joy while preparing a plant-based menu.

**Response modulation** involves making changes to maximise the impact of an experience through the actions we take. For instance, it could mean telling your partner how much you enjoy the comedy gig or discussing the funniest jokes during intermission. While running in the park you may modulate your response to the positive experiences by smiling to passers-by. Or when preparing a menu you may choose to add a social component by involving your entire family in the joyful process.

The Positive Emotion Regulation process (Quoidbach et al., 2015) is, therefore, a tool that optimises positive outcomes in various situations. It is applicable to both positive and negative experiences. For instance, consider a disagreement with a colleague at work, though this may initially be upsetting. To apply the Positive Emotion Regulation process in this situation, you might seize the opportunity to openly discuss the disagreement, and then modify the situation by reflecting on the positive intentions behind both perspectives. During the discussion, attentional deployment allows you to observe your and your colleagues' emotions, behaviours, and facial expressions. This may prompt a shift in thinking about the situation and instead of seeking retaliation, you might focus on forgiveness. Alternatively, rather than dwelling on hurt feelings, you might consider how the argument has strengthened your workplace relationship. Finally, in response to modulation, you can express these reconciliatory thoughts in a way that fosters improved relationships going forward. Therefore, this model can be used not only to amplify positive experiences but also to neutralise negative ones in our lives. Given its overall positive impact on our wellbeing, it could also serve as a powerful tool in promoting lifestyle changes during a positive health journey.

In positive health, these experiences could involve attempts to quit smoking, combat drug abuse, or reduce excessive alcohol consumption. Alternatively, it may entail reframing how we perceive our bodies during weight loss journeys. Rather than dwelling on negatives and avoidance tactics, this approach could allow us to focus on positives and explore avenues for growth. Consider the potential benefits this could offer your practice. Similarly, delving into motivations using this framework could accelerate progress when encountering challenges in maintaining physical activity. Thus, this method could serve as a valuable tool for fostering positive health outcomes, although further research is required to assess its effectiveness in this domain.

## MAKING POSITIVE HEALTH CHANGES

The Transtheoretical Model of Change, one of the main models in lifestyle medicine, was proposed by Prochaska et al. (1997). This model, provides a crucial framework for individuals embarking on lifestyle modifications, outlining five distinct stages:

**Pre-contemplation**: At this stage, individuals are oblivious to the need for change. They have not yet recognised the potential benefits of altering their lifestyle habits.

**Contemplation**: In this phase, individuals acknowledge that change may be necessary but are still contemplating whether to commit to it. They weigh the pros and cons and assess their readiness for change.

**Preparation**: Individuals are primed to take concrete steps toward change as they progress to the preparation stage. They are actively planning and preparing for the adjustments they need to make.

**Action**: The action stage marks the commencement of specific efforts to implement change. In this phase, individuals modify their behaviours and habits to align with their health goals.

**Maintenance and relapse**: After successfully initiating change, individuals enter the maintenance stage, where they strive to sustain their new habits over the long term. However, relapses may occur, prompting individuals to revisit earlier stages of the model. This understanding and support in revisiting earlier stages are crucial as they work to regain their momentum and commitment to their positive health journey.

When exploring the Transtheoretical Model of Change, it is important to recognise the dynamic nature of behaviour change and the need for tailored interventions at each stage of the process. By understanding where individuals are in their journey toward healthy lifestyle changes, practitioners can provide targeted support and resources to facilitate progress. Additionally, emphasising the potential for relapse could offer them ongoing supports and strategies for resilience. These are crucial to maintaining outcomes over time, providing a safety net in the face of challenges.

## Agnieszka's journey

*In the heart of Poland, lived a woman named Agnieszka. For years, alcohol has become her loyal companion, her solace in moments of joy and sorrow. Yet, as the toll on her health became evident, Agnieszka knew it was time to quit drinking.*

*Agnieszka acknowledged the need for change and signed up to an Alcohol Anonymous (AA) group. There she met new people who became her support in the times of despair. While she initially progressed well, a few weeks into her journey she went out with her old friends and ten drinks later, she found herself lying on a street unable to get up.*

*She was disappointed with herself but went back to AA the following day. There she learnt about the transtheoretical model of change and became aware that relapse was a natural part of the change process. With each relapse, she learned valuable lessons about her triggers and vulnerabilities, using this knowledge to fortify her resolve.*

The process of making positive change is intricate and involves both cognitive and emotional shifts. It incorporates various tools aimed at guiding individuals along the path of change. These tools encompass strategies like counterconditioning, experiencing emotional relief, and re-evaluating one's environment. For instance, consider the challenge of improving sleep habits. Initially, an individual may be oblivious to the extent of their sleep debt, unaware that their sleeping patterns pose an issue. However, once they acknowledge this issue, they may begin contemplating change, seeking guidance from a positive health coach. Over time, they embark on a transformation journey, implementing a repertoire of sleep-enhancing techniques learned through positive health coaching.

This process is also used within positive psychology, yet the positive psychology goals we establish for ourselves are significant and can potentially help or hinder the process of change and outcomes. It is beneficial to view happiness or wellbeing as a by-product of a fulfilling life journey. Researchers caution against solely pursuing it as an objective, as this approach may lead to a realisation of dissatisfaction with life, resulting in a further decline in wellbeing or heightened loneliness due to excessive focus on this positive outcome (Mauss et al., 2011, 2012). This is why some scholars advocate for emphasising positivity as a goal instead (Hansenne et al., 2021), wherein the focus shifts to the process rather than solely fixating on the result, such as happiness. Hence, the Transtheoretical Model of Change can be employed in positive psychology wellbeing plans to enhance positivity or specific aspects of wellbeing, like cultivating optimistic thinking or increasing engagement with life; however, it also needs to be used with caution.

Given that the Transtheoretical Model of Change is used across various fields of social sciences, this model could also be applied to promote positive health outcomes in individuals. However, the need for future research to delve deeper into the outcomes of positive health are important. If prioritising happiness impacts wellbeing negatively, it's important to investigate whether emphasising specific facets of positive health might yield similar adverse effects. For instance, when assisting individuals post-heart attack, awaiting a liver transplant, or elderly people grappling with multiple ailments, what interventions should take precedence? Should we focus on lifestyle behaviours or wellbeing-inductive thoughts? Furthermore, how do we gauge success when confronted with age-related health decline? What constitutes the optimal balance between positive psychology and lifestyle medicine approaches to bolster individuals navigating diverse health conditions? Addressing these questions is crucial for advancing research in positive health.

Finally, most modifications within lifestyle medicine revolve around altering behaviours. Conversely, positive psychology places significant emphasis on shifting emotions and thoughts. Behavioural strategies relate to positive psychology interventions, focusing on cultivating habits to help individuals practice them regularly. It's important to determine the factors that impact the implementation of positive health. Consequently, while change within positive health appears straightforward, it is in fact, intricately complex, currently raising more questions than providing answers.

## APPLYING POSITIVE HEALTH IN DAILY LIFE

The Person–Activity Fit Model (Lyubomirsky & Layous, 2013) emphasises the importance of tailoring positive psychology interventions to individual characteristics and preferences. This model recognises that the effectiveness of such activities varies based on personal differences, including personality traits, values, interests, and current life circumstances. Activities, such as gratitude practices, acts of kindness, savouring, optimism exercises, mindfulness, and goal setting are more effective when they align with what individuals naturally enjoy and find meaningful in life. By focusing on activities that fit well with an individual's unique profile, the model aims to increase the likelihood of sustained engagement and positive outcomes.

Implementing the Person–Activity Fit Model empowers individuals by allowing them to take control of their wellbeing. It starts with an initial assessment of their traits and preferences, using a diagnostic tool, followed by the selection of a few suitable interventions. This personalised approach aims to enhance the overall engagement and effectiveness of positive psychology interventions, leading to more significant improvements in wellbeing, increased happiness, reduced stress, and better mental health.

In contrast to the predominant focus on intervention strategies in research, our recent investigation into positive psychology demonstrates an interesting trend. According to Burke and Giraldez-Hayes (2023), individuals versed in the science of wellbeing don't practice positive psychology interventions according to the guidelines in the Person–Activity Fit model. Initially, as they embark on their positive psychology journey, they embrace positive psychology interventions and practice wellbeing activities regularly. However, as they progress, they integrate the principles of positive psychology seamlessly into their daily lives. Therefore, they do not sit down once a day to savour eating an apple as part of their wellbeing plan; instead, they slow down and savour their food at all meals, or make music part of their life and start a day by putting it on, or they create some "me" time throughout the day during which they do what they love. In other words, they make informed wellbeing choices on integrating flourishing interventions into their lifestyle. This is the ultimate practice of positive health – integrating wellbeing and health practices in our daily lives.

## SUMMARY

This chapter delved into the transformative impact of positive health on overall mental health by integrating wellbeing models into lifestyle changes. It highlighted the significant benefits the positive health approach offers to health and overall quality of life. By incorporating elements such as positive emotions, flow experiences, a sense of life purpose, and nurturing positive relationships, individuals can enhance their wellbeing, which will help them experience flourishing regardless of their health status or a stage of a journey towards healthier lifestyle.

However, the chapter also highlighted the necessity of a more integrated approach. It emphasised the importance of future research and practice in considering not only the success of lifestyle changes but also their impact on mental health. This holistic perspective acknowledges the intricate interplay between physical health, mental health, and lifestyle choices. By adopting a comprehensive approach that accounts for both the physical and mental dimensions of health, individuals can optimise their wellbeing and foster lasting positive change in their lives.

## REFERENCES

Carpentier, J., Mageau, G. A., & Vallerand, R. J. (2012). Ruminations and flow: Why do people with a more harmonious passion experience higher wellbeing?. *Journal of Happiness Studies, 13*, 501–518. https://doi.org/10.1007/s10902-011-9276-4

Catalino, L. I., & Fredrickson, B. L. (2011). A Tuesday in the life of a flourisher: The role of positive emotional reactivity in optimal mental health. *Emotion, 11*(4), 938–950. https://doi.org/10.1037/a0024889

Cohen, S., Doyle, W. J., Turner, R. B., Alper, C. M., & Skoner, D. P. (2003). Emotional style and susceptibility to the common cold. *Psychosomatic Medicine, 65*(4), 652–657. https://doi.org/10.1097/01.psy.0000077508.57784.da

Conradson, H. E., Hayden, K. A., Russell, M. S., Raffin Bouchal, S., & King, S. K. (2022). Positive psychological well-being in women with obesity: A scoping review of qualitative and quantitative primary research. *Obesity Science & Practice*, *8*(6), 691–714. https://doi.org/10.1002/osp4.605

Brennan, F. X., & Charnetski, C. J. (2000). Explanatory style and Immunoglobulin A (IgA). *Integrative Physiological & Behavioral Science*, *35*(4), 251–255. https://doi.org/10.1007/BF02688787

Brown, N. J., Sokal, A. D., & Friedman, H. L. (2013). The complex dynamics of wishful thinking: The critical positivity ratio. *The American Psychologist*, *68*(9), 801–813. https://doi.org/10.1037/a0032850

Burke, J., & Dunne, P.J. (2024). Mind meets body: Lifestyle medicine and positive psychology interventions for school. In G. Arslan & M. Yildirim (Eds.), *Handbook of positive school psychology interventions: Evidence-based practice for promoting youth mental health*. Springer.

Burke, J., & Giraldez-Hayes, A. (2023). The sustained wellbeing model: Insights from the MAPP alumni on how to sustain wellbeing. [poster presentation]. IPPA World Congress on Positive Psychology, Vancouver, Canada. www.vancouverconventioncentre.com/events/ippa-world-congress-on-positive-psychology

Burton, C. M., & King, L. A. (2004). The health benefits of writing about intensely positive experiences. *Journal of Research in Personality*, *38*, 150–163. https://doi.org/10.1016/S0092-6566(03)00058-8

Curry, O. S., Rowland, L. A., Van Lissa, C. J., Zlotowitz, S., McAlaney, J., & Whitehouse, H. (2018). Happy to help? A systematic review and meta-analysis of the effects of performing acts of kindness on the well-being of the actor. *Journal of Experimental Social Psychology*, *76*, 320–329. https://doi.org/10.1016/j.jesp.2018.02.014

Dahlen, M., & Thorbjørnsen, H. (2022). An infectious silver lining: Is there a positive relationship between recovering from a COVID infection and psychological richness of life?. *Frontiers in Psychology*, *13*, 785224. https://doi.org/10.3389/fpsyg.2022.785224

Decloe, M. D., Kaczynski, A. T., & Havitz, M. E. (2009). Social participation, flow and situational involvement in recreational physical activity. *Journal of Leisure Research*, *41*, 73–90. https://doi.org/10.1080/00222216.2009.11950160

Diener, E. (1984). Subjective well-being. *Psychological Bulletin*, *95*, 542–575.

Diener, E., Wirtz, D., Tov, W., Kim-Prieto, C., Choi, D., Oishi, S., & Biswas-Diener, R. (2009). New measures of wellbeing: Flourishing and positive and negative feelings. *Social Indicators Research*, *39*, 247–266.

Diener, E., Oishi, S., & Tay, L. (2018). Advances in subjective well-being research. *Nature Human Behaviour*, *2*(4), 253–260. https://doi.org/10.1038/s41562-018-0307-6

Ekman, P. (1992). An argument for basic emotions. *Cognition and Emotion*, 6(3–4), 169–200. https://doi.org/10.1080/02699939208411068

Elbe, A. M., Strahler, K., Krustrup, P., Wikman, J., & Stelter, R. (2010). Experiencing flow in different types of physical activity intervention programs: Three randomized studies. *Scandinavian Journal of Medicine & Science in Sports*, 20(Suppl 1), 111–117. https://doi.org/10.1111/j.1600-0838.2010.01112.x

Emmons, R. A., & McCullough, M. E. (2003). Counting blessings versus burdens: An experimental investigation of gratitude and subjective well-being in daily life. *Journal of Personality and Social Psychology*, 84(2), 377–389. https://doi.org/10.1037/0022-3514.84.2.377

Fantini, L., Gostoli, S., Artin, M. G., & Rafanelli, C. (2024). An intervention based on Well-Being Therapy to prevent alcohol use and other unhealthy lifestyle behaviors among students: A three-arm cluster randomized controlled trial. *Psychology, Health & Medicine*, 29(5), 930–950. https://doi.org/10.1080/13548506.2023.2235740

Fernet, C., Lavigne, G. L., Vallerand, R. J., & Austin, S. (2014). Fired up with passion: Investigating how job autonomy and passion predict burnout at career start in teachers. *Work & Stress*, 28(3), 270–288. https://doi.org/10.1080/02678373.2014.935524

Fowler, J. H., & Christakis, N. A. (2008). Dynamic spread of happiness in a large social network: Longitudinal analysis over 20 years in the Framingham Heart Study. *British Medical Journal* (Clinical research ed.), 337, a2338. https://doi.org/10.1136/bmj.a2338

Fredrickson, B. L. (2001). The role of positive emotions in positive psychology. The broaden-and-build theory of positive emotions. *The American Psychologist*, 56(3), 218–226. https://doi.org/10.1037/0003-066x.56.3.218

Fredrickson, B. L., & Losada, M. F. (2005). Positive affect and the complex dynamics of human flourishing. *American Psychologist*, 60(7), 678–686. https://doi.org/10.1037/0003-066X.60.7.678

Gable, S. L., Reis, H. T., Impett, E. A., & Asher, E. R. (2004). What do you do when things go right? The intrapersonal and interpersonal benefits of sharing positive events. *Journal of Personality and Social Psychology*, 87(2), 228–245. https://doi.org/10.1037/0022-3514.87.2.228

Gander, F., Proyer, R. T., Ruch, W., & Wyss, T. (2013). Strength-based positive interventions: Further evidence for their potential in enhancing well-being and alleviating depression. *Journal of Happiness Studies: An Interdisciplinary Forum on Subjective Well-Being*, 14(4), 1241–1259. https://doi.org/10.1007/s10902-012-9380-0

Gibson, B., Umeh, K., Davies, I., & Newson, L. (2021). The best possible self-intervention as a viable public health tool for the prevention of type 2 diabetes: A reflexive thematic analysis of public experience and engagement.

*Health Expectations: An International Journal of Public Participation in Health Care and Health Policy, 24*(5), 1713–1724. https://doi.org/10.1111/hex.13311

Gostoli, S., Fantini, L., Casadei, S., De Angelis, V. A., & Rafanelli, C. (2021). Binge drinking in 14-year-old Italian students is correlated with low or high psychological wellbeing: A cross-sectional study. *Drugs: Education, Prevention & Policy, 28*(2), 190–199. https://doi.org/10.1080/09687637.2020.1799942

Gottman, J. (2000). *The seven principles for making marriage work.* Orion.

Gu, Y., Tao, L., & Zheng, W. (2023). Relationship between COVID-19-related stress and social inhibition among university students in China: The mediating role of psychological richness. *Social and Personality Psychology Compass, 17*(11), Article e12872. https://doi.org/10.1111/spc3.12872

Hansenne, M. (2021). Valuing happiness is not a good way of pursuing happiness, but prioritizing positivity is: A replication study. *Psychologica Belgica, 61*(1), 315–326. https://doi.org/10.5334/pb.1036

Heintzelman, S. J., & King, L. A. (2014). Life is pretty meaningful. *American Psychologist, 69*(6), 561–574. https://doi.org/10.1037/a0035049

Hicks, J. A., & King, L. A. (2009). Positive mood and social relatedness as information about meaning in life. *The Journal of Positive Psychology, 4*(6), 471–482. https://doi.org/10.1080/17439760903271108

Hoemann, K., Barrett, L. F., & Quigley, K. S. (2021). Emotional granularity increases with intensive ambulatory assessment: Methodological and individual factors influence how much. *Frontiers in Psychology, 12*, 704125. https://doi.org/10.3389/fpsyg.2021.704125

Huppert, F. A., & So, T. T. (2013). Flourishing across Europe: Application of a new conceptual framework for defining well-being. *Social Indicators Research, 110*(3), 837–861. https://doi.org/10.1007/s11205-011-9966-7

Ikeda, S. (2023). The more emotional words you know, the higher your mental health. *Scandinavian Journal of Psychology, 64*(6), 705–709. https://doi.org/10.1111/sjop.12928

Isen, A. M. (1999). Positive affect. In T. Dalgleish & M. J. Power (Eds.), *Handbook of cognition and emotion* (pp. 521–539). John Wiley. https://doi.org/10.1002/0470013494.ch25

Jamieson, J. P., Crum, A. J., Goyer, J. P., Marotta, M. E., & Akinola, M. (2018). Optimizing stress responses with reappraisal and mindset interventions: An integrated model. *Anxiety, Stress, and Coping, 31*(3), 245–261. https://doi.org/10.1080/10615806.2018.1442615

Kamen-Siegel, L., Rodin, J., Seligman, M. E., & Dwyer, J. (1991). Explanatory style and cell-mediated immunity in elderly men and women. *Health Psychology, 10*(4), 229–235. https://doi.org/10.1037/0278-6133.10.4.229

Kahneman, D., & Riis, J. (2005). Living, and thinking about it: two perspectives on life. In F. A. Huppert, N. Baylis, & B. Keverne (Eds.), *The science of well-being* (pp. 285–304). Oxford University Press. https://doi.org/10.1093/acprof:oso/9780198567523.003.0011

Kashdan, T. B., Barrett, L. F., & McKnight, P. E. (2015). Unpacking emotion differentiation: Transforming unpleasant experience by perceiving distinctions in negativity. *Current Directions in Psychological Science, 24*(1), 10–16. https://doi.org/10.1177/0963721414550708

Keyes, C. L. M. (2002). The mental health continuum: From languishing to flourishing in life. *Journal of Health and Social Behavior, 43*(2), 207–222. https://doi.org/10.2307/3090197

Kiely, B., Croke, A., O'Shea, M., Boland, F., O'Shea, E., Connolly, D., & Smith, S. M. (2022). Effect of social prescribing link workers on health outcomes and costs for adults in primary care and community settings: A systematic review. *British Medical Journal open, 12*(10), e062951. https://doi.org/10.1136/bmjopen-2022-062951

King, L. A., & Miner, K. N. (2000). Writing about the perceived benefits of traumatic events: Implications for physical health. *Personality and Social Psychology Bulletin, 26*(2), 220–230. https://doi.org/10.1177/0146167200264008

Ko, K., Margolis, S., Revord, J., & Lyubomirsky, S. (2019). Comparing the effects of performing and recalling acts of kindness. *Journal of Positive Psychology, 16*(1), 73–81. https://doi.org/10.1080/17439760.2019.1663252

Li, C. H. (2010). Predicting subjective vitality and performance in sports: The role of passion and achievement goals. *Perceptual and Motor Skills, 110*(3 Pt 2), 1029–1047. https://doi.org/10.2466/pms.110.C.1029-1047

Li, J.-B., Dou, K., & Liang, Y. (2021). The relationship between presence of meaning, search for meaning, and subjective well-being: A three-level meta-analysis based on the Meaning in Life Questionnaire. *Journal of Happiness Studies: An Interdisciplinary Forum on Subjective Well-Being, 22*(1), 467–489. https://doi.org/10.1007/s10902-020-00230-y

Lianov, L. S., Fredrickson, B. L., Barron, C., Krishnaswami, J., & Wallace, A. (2019). Positive psychology in lifestyle medicine and health care: Strategies for Implementation. *American Journal of Lifestyle Medicine, 13*(5), 480–486. https://doi.org/10.1177/1559827619838992

Lin, C-F., Lo, K-Y., Su, Y-J., Kao, H-F., Lin, I-T., Ho, C-C., Shieh, J-C., & Lee, P-F. (2023). Associations of self-reported happiness with body mass index and obesity risks among young adults in Taiwan. PREPRINT (Version 1) Research Square. https://doi.org/10.21203/rs.3.rs-2864752/v1

Lincoln, K. D., Chatters, L. M., Taylor, R. J. (2003). Psychological distress among black and white Americans: Differential effects of social support, negative interaction and personal control. *Journal of Health and Social Behavior, 44*(3), 390–407.

Liu, Y., Xu, L., & Hagedorn, A. (2022). How is obesity associated with happiness? Evidence from China. *Journal of Health Psychology, 27*(3), 568–580. https://doi.org/10.1177/1359105320962268

Lyubomirsky, S., King, L., & Diener, E. (2005). The benefits of frequent positive affect: Does happiness lead to success? *Psychological Bulletin, 131*(6), 803–855. https://doi.org/10.1037/0033-2909.131.6.803

Lyubomirsky, S., & Layous, K. (2013). How do simple positive activities increase well-being? *Current Directions in Psychological Science, 22*(1), 57–62. https://doi.org/10.1177/0963721412469809

Majeed, N. M., Lua, V. Y. Q., Chong, J. S., Lew, Z., & Hartanto, A. (2021). Does bedtime music listening improve subjective sleep quality and next-morning wellbeing in young adults? A randomized cross-over trial. *Psychomusicology: Music, Mind and Brain, 31*(3–4), 149–158. https://doi.org/10.1037/pmu0000283

Major, B. C., Le Nguyen, K. D., Lundberg, K. B., & Fredrickson, B. L. (2018). Well-being correlates of perceived positivity resonance: Evidence from trait and episode-level assessments. *Personality & Social Psychology Bulletin, 44*(12), 1631–1647. https://doi.org/10.1177/0146167218771324

Mauss, I. B., Tamir, M., Anderson, C. L., & Savino, N. S. (2011). Can seeking happiness make people unhappy? Paradoxical effects of valuing happiness. *Emotion, 11*(4), 807–815. https://doi.org/10.1037/a0022010

Mauss, I. B., Savino, N. S., Anderson, C. L., Weisbuch, M., Tamir, M., & Laudenslager, M. L. (2012). The pursuit of happiness can be lonely. *Emotion, 12*(5), 908–912. https://doi.org/10.1037/a0025299

Morton, D. P. (2018). Combining lifestyle medicine and positive psychology to improve mental health and emotional well-being. *American Journal of Lifestyle Medicine. 12*(5), 370–374. doi:10.1177/1559827618766482

Nelson, S. K., Layous, K., Cole, S. W., & Lyubomirsky, S. (2016). Do unto others or treat yourself? The effects of prosocial and self-focused behavior on psychological flourishing. *Emotion, 16*(6), 850–861. https://doi.org/10.1037/emo0000178

Oishi, S., & Westgate, E. C. (2022). A psychologically rich life: Beyond happiness and meaning. *Psychological Review, 129*(4), 790–811. https://doi.org/10.1037/rev0000317

Pennebaker, J. W., & Francis, M. E. (1996). Cognitive, emotional, and language processes in disclosure. *Cognition and Emotion, 10*(6), 601–626. https://doi.org/10.1080/026999396380079

Peterson, C. (2013). *Pursuing the good life: 100 reflections on positive psychology.* Oxford University Press.

Pressman, S. D., Jenkins, B. N., & Moskowitz, J. T. (2019). Positive affect and health: What do we know and where next should we go? *Annual Review of Psychology, 70,* 627–650. https://doi.org/10.1146/annurev-psych-010418-102955

Prochaska, J. O., & Velicer, W. F. (1997). The transtheoretical model of health behavior change. *American Journal of Health Promotion, 12*(1), 38–48. https://doi.org/10.4278/0890-1171-12.1.38

Provine, R.R. (2000). *Laughter: A scientific investigation.* Penguin.

Przybylko, G., Morton, D., Kent, L., Morton, J., Hinze, J., Beamish, P., & Renfrew, M. (2021). The effectiveness of an online interdisciplinary intervention for mental health promotion: A randomized controlled trial. *BMC Psychology, 9*(77). https://doi.org/10.1186/s40359-021-00577-8

Quoidbach, J., Mikolajczak, M., & Gross, J. J. (2015). Positive interventions: An emotion regulation perspective. *Psychological Bulletin, 141*(3), 655–693. https://doi.org/10.1037/a0038648

Rand, K., Vallis, M., Aston, M., Price, S., Piccinini-Vallis, H., Rehman, L., & Kirk, S. F. L. (2017). "It is not the diet; it is the mental part we need help with." A multilevel analysis of psychological, emotional, and social wellbeing in obesity. *International Journal of Qualitative Studies on Health and Wellbeing, 12*(1), 1306421. https://doi.org/10.1080/17482631.2017.1306421

Reker, G. T., & Wong, P. T. P. (1988). Aging as an individual process: Toward a theory of personal meaning. In J. E. Birren & V. L. Bengtson (Eds.), *Emergent theories of aging* (pp. 214–246). Springer.

Roepke, A. M., Jayawickreme, E., & Riffle, O. M. (2014). Meaning and health: A systematic review. *Applied Research in Quality of Life, 9*(4), 1055–1079. https://doi.org/10.1007/s11482-013-9288-9

Ryan, R. M., & Deci, E. L. (2000). Self-determination theory and the facilitation of intrinsic motivation, social development, and well-being. *American Psychologist, 55*(1), 68–78. https://doi.org/10.1037/0003-066X.55.1.68

Ryff, C. D. (1995). Psychological well-being in adult life. *Current Directions in Psychological Science, 4*(4), 99–104. https://doi.org/10.1111/1467-8721.ep10772395

Ryff, C. D., & Singer, B. (1998). The contours of positive human health. *Psychological Inquiry, 9*(1), 1–28. https://doi.org/10.1207/s15327965pli0901_1

Scheier, M. F., Matthews, K. A., Owens, J. F., Magovern, G. J., Sr, Lefebvre, R. C., Abbott, R. A., & Carver, C. S. (1989). Dispositional optimism and recovery from coronary artery bypass surgery: The beneficial effects on physical and psychological well-being. *Journal of Personality and Social Psychology, 57*(6), 1024–1040. https://doi.org/10.1037//0022-3514.57.6.1024

Schellenberg, B. J., Gaudreau, P., & Crocker, P. R. (2013). Passion and coping: Relationships with changes in burnout and goal attainment in collegiate volleyball players. *Journal of Sport & Exercise Psychology, 35*(3), 270–280. https://doi.org/10.1123/jsep.35.3.270

Schmidt, C., Häggström, M. (2022). We are alive and thus need to belong, participate, and act!. In M. Häggström & C. Schmidt (Eds.), *Relational and critical perspectives on education for sustainable development.* Sustainable Development Goals Series. Springer. https://doi.org/10.1007/978-3-030-84510-0_12

Seligman, M. E. P. (1975). *Helplessness: On depression, development, and death.* W. H. Freeman/Times Books/Henry Holt & Co.

Seligman, M. E. P. (1998). *Learned optimism.* Pocket Books.

Seligman, M. E. P. (2002). *Authentic happiness: Using the new positive psychology to realize your potential for lasting fulfillment.* Free Press.

Seligman, M. E. P. (2011). *Flourish: A visionary new understanding of happiness and well-being.* Free Press.

Stavrou, N. A. M., Psychountaki, M., Georgiadis, E., Karteroliotis, K., & Zervas, Y. (2015). Flow theory–goal orientation theory: Positive experience is related to athlete's goal orientation. *Frontiers in Psychology, 6,* 1499. https://doi.org/10.3389/fpsyg.2015.01499

Steger, M. F. (2012). Experiencing meaning in life: Optimal functioning at the nexus of well-being, psychopathology, and spirituality. In P. T. P. Wong (Ed.), *The human quest for meaning: Theories, research, and applications* (2nd ed., pp. 165–184). Routledge.

Steger, M. F. (2017). Meaning in life and wellbeing. In M. Slade, L. Oades, & A. Jarden (Eds.), *Wellbeing, recovery and mental health* (pp. 75–85). Cambridge University Press. https://doi.org/10.1017/9781316339275.008

Steger, M. F., Shim, Y., Barenz, J., & Shin, J. Y. (2014). Through the windows of the soul: A pilot study using photography to enhance meaning in life. *Journal of Contextual Behavioral Science, 3*(1), 27–30. https://doi.org/10.1016/j.jcbs.2013.11.002

Stein, N., Folkman, S., Trabasso, T., & Richards, T. A. (1997). Appraisal and goal processes as predictors of psychological well-being in bereaved caregivers. *Journal of Personality and Social Psychology, 72*(4), 872–884. https://doi.org/10.1037//0022-3514.72.4.872

Vaillant, G. E., & Mukamal, K. (2001). Successful aging. *The American Journal of Psychiatry, 158*(6), 839–847. https://doi.org/10.1176/appi.ajp.158.6.839

Vallerand, R. J., Blanchard, C., Mageau, G. A., Koestner, R., Ratelle, C., Léonard, M., Gagné, M., & Marsolais, J. (2003). Les passions de l'âme: On obsessive and harmonious passion. *Journal of Personality and Social Psychology, 85*(4), 756–767. https://doi.org/10.1037/0022-3514.85.4.756

Vallerand, R. J., Salvy, S. J., Mageau, G. A., Elliot, A. J., Denis, P. L., Grouzet, F. M., & Blanchard, C. (2007). On the role of passion in performance. *Journal of Personality*, *75*(3), 505–533. https://doi.org/10.1111/j.1467-6494.2007.00447

Werner, E. E. (1993). Risk, resilience, and recovery: Perspectives from the Kauai Longitudinal Study. *Development and Psychopathology*, *5*(4), 503–515. https://doi.org/10.1017/S095457940000612X

Wong, P. T. P. (2011). Positive psychology 2.0: Towards a balanced interactive model of the good life. *Canadian Psychology / Psychologie canadienne*, *52*(2), 69–81. https://doi.org/10.1037/a0022511

Zhu, B., Gostoli, S., Benasi, G., Patierno, C., Petroni, M. L., Nuccitelli, C., Marchesini, G., Fava, G. A., & Rafanelli, C. (2022). The role of psychological well-being in weight loss: New Insights from a comprehensive lifestyle intervention. *International Journal of Clinical and Health Psychology*, *22*(1), 100279. https://doi.org/10.1016/j.ijchp.2021.100279

# 3

# POSITIVE HEALTH IN MENTAL HEALTH STRUGGLES

What differentiates positive health from other approaches is its focus not only on helping healthy individuals improve their wellbeing, but also assisting those who have mental health issues and other type of illness or disease to enhance their wellbeing regardless of their health. In this chapter we will explore some of the existing research about ways in which positive health can assist individuals with mental health conditions.

*Please note that this chapter is written with the mental health professionals in mind, not their patients, to allow them to explore positive health approaches that exist for mental disorders. It is of utmost importance that anyone experiencing mental health conditions consults a healthcare professional before attempting any of the activities in this book.*

Positive health approaches can be beneficial for many mental health conditions. This includes exploring the flourishing levels of individuals experiencing mental health issues and trying interventions from positive psychology and lifestyle medicine that may reduce symptoms or improve wellbeing. In general, flourishing effectively prevents mental health conditions, reducing mood disorders by 27% and anxiety disorders by 53% (Schotanus–Dijkstra et al., 2017). However, mental health conditions and flourishing are not always correlated; individuals may experience high levels of flourishing while coping with mental health issues. This also indicates that individuals with mental health conditions can live a good life and even flourish despite their conditions.

DOI: 10.4324/9781003457169-3

## DEPRESSION AND ANXIETY

Positive psychology research and interventions have been extensively tested with individuals experiencing depression and anxiety.
The founder of Positive Psychology, Prof. Marty Seligman, specialised in depression research for decades before his contributions to
positive psychology. Consequently, the impact of interventions on
anxiety and depression has been his focus from the outset.

The encouraging news is that individuals with depression or
anxiety can still experience flourishing. Research involving over
20,000 participants found that 39% of those previously diagnosed
with depression experienced psychological flourishing (Fuller-
Thompson et al., 2016). Factors such as strong social support,
mainly through marriage or significant relationships, along with
effective coping strategies, religion, and spirituality associated
with finding meaning in life, and regular exercise, contribute to
their flourishing (Corrigan & Phelan, 2004; Westerhof & Keyes,
2010; Daley, 2008; Dein, 2006). Unfortunately, socio–economic
status plays a role in future flourishing prospects for individuals
with depression, with lower-income individuals less likely to attain
complete mental health (Gilmour, 2014). This disparity could stem
from limited access to beneficial interventions or other environmental factors hindering optimal levels of wellbeing. Thus, while
some factors are within individuals' control, others are influenced
by external circumstances.

### Daniel's journey

*Daniel Harper's early life was turbulent, marked by his parents' men-
tal health struggles – his father was diagnosed with severe depression,
and his mother with anxiety. His childhood was filled with worries
and struggle.*

*From a young age, Daniel felt very anxious. As he entered young
adulthood, the weight of anxiety continued to grow. The pressures of
college and the uncertainty of his future felt overwhelming, leading
Daniel to seek therapy. Therapy helped him unravel his thoughts
and manage anxiety more effectively, but he still felt like something
was missing.*

*Daniel immersed himself in self-help books, workshops, and online communities and began to explore the new science of positive health. He discovered he was a highly sensitive person, which explained his intense reactions to events that didn't seem to bother his peers. He began hiking and met a group of like-minded people who enjoyed exploring mountain tops every weekend. They became his companions and witnesses to his deepening connection with nature, bringing about feelings of transcendence which he had never experienced before. His love for nature inspired him to set up a travel company that helped others connect with the outdoors at a deeper level. This became his life's purpose – to help others discover the healing properties of nature.*

*Daniel transformed from barely managing his daily anxieties to feeling fulfilled, purposeful, and content within a decade. He finally felt like his life mattered; he mattered; and what he did for others mattered.*

## INTERVENTIONS

A recent systematic review and meta-analysis (Carr et al., 2021) demonstrated that interventions such as savouring and forgiveness significantly reduced symptoms of depression. Other interventions, such as goal setting, practising optimism, hope, humour, gratitude, exploring meaning-making, and using personal strengths, had a moderate impact on wellbeing, while other interventions showed only a small effect.

Also, interventions such as expressive writing mentioned earlier, practising forgiveness, savouring, and humour were the most effective interventions for reducing anxiety. Meaning-making, optimism, and hope were moderately effective, with other interventions having a negligible impact. These findings offer hope to all those who experience anxiety or depression, as engaging in positive activities could help them navigate their symptoms with more ease and support them on their journey.

Below, you will find examples of interventions from each category presented in this systematic review. Note that some studies assessed clinical patients, while others evaluated the general population with undiagnosed symptoms of anxiety and depression.

## LETTER FROM THE FUTURE

### (Hoffman et al., 2010)

Write to your current self from your future self, outlining key goals and the strategies you used to achieve them, so that you can experience your desired life. Ensure goals are challenging yet achievable. They need to resonate with your personal values and hold significance to you. They also need to have clear criteria that allows you to track your progress towards achieving them. In your writing, make sure you take time to celebrate your future accomplishments, which will allow you to experience a stronger belief that they could happen and drive your motivation towards making them happen.

### Letter of forgiveness (adapted from Worthington et al., 2000)

Take the next 30 minutes to compose a letter to someone who wronged you. In the letter, (a) provide a brief overview of the incident; (b) share your understanding of the offender's motives; (c) explain your reasons for desiring forgiveness; and (d) explicitly state your forgiveness towards the individual who caused you harm or offence.

### Savouring past events (Biskas et al., 2019)

Recall a past positive experience involving others, such as school friendships or meeting your partner. Reflect on the situations you have recalled and emotions you had experienced. Try to describe your memory in four words. Then, dedicate 5–10 minutes to writing down or reflecting upon the details of your experience and its emotional impact.

### Humour (adapted from Wellenzohn et al., 2016)

After encountering a stressful situation, take time to reflect on it, considering how you could have resolved it with humour. At the end of the day, sit down and consider the humorous moments you had experienced and brainstorm ways to incorporate more laughter into the next day.

**Hope profiling (adapted from Lopez et al., 2004)**

Write five stories detailing past or present goal pursuits, including how the goals were developed, paths followed, and motivations. Create a table with three columns: "Goals", "Pathways", and "Obstacles", under "Goals", list a goal using one of your strengths. In the "Pathways" column, outline at least three ways to achieve the goal or use your personal strengths. In the "Obstacles" column, note at least one obstacle for each pathway. Reflect on maintaining motivation by identifying supportive individuals and additional resources.

**Through the windows of the soul (Steger et al., 2014)**

For the next week, keep a camera or your smartphone handy. Capture 9–12 photos of what brings meaning to your life, be it the sunrise, or the people you love. After a week, reflect on each photo, noting what it represents and why you find it meaningful.

Another extensive analysis, encompassing over half a million participants, revealed that even slight to moderate reductions in depression and anxiety had lasting effects, with participants maintaining improved wellbeing up to 7.5 months later (Carr et al., 2024). Interestingly, mind–body interventions referred to in this book as positive health Interventions, such as yoga, demonstrated significant efficacy. This study highlights the profound influence of positive health practices on depression and overall wellbeing.

Regarding anxiety, positive psychology interventions have evidence of effectiveness not only in reducing anxiety among non-clinical individuals but also in those diagnosed with anxiety disorders (Brown et al., 2019). Although the magnitude of change was modest to moderate, interventions delivered by healthcare professionals yielded better results than self-administered ones. Additionally, longer-duration interventions proved more effective than shorter ones, emphasising the importance of careful intervention design. These findings provide some guidance on how to optimise the impact of positive activities on individuals diagnosed with anxiety.

A similar trend emerged regarding lifestyle medicine. Meta-analytic studies indicated that lifestyle medicine interventions effectively reduced anxiety and depression, but this effect was observed only immediately post-intervention (Wong et al., 2021, 2022). Once more, interventions incorporating multiple components proved more effective. Considering the short-term impact of lifestyle medicine interventions, there's potential for combining lifestyle medicine and positive psychology interventions into positive health interventions to yield a particularly powerful effect. Nonetheless, future research should delve into this area to evaluate their medium and long-term impacts.

## POST-TRAUMATIC STRESS DISORDER

Post-traumatic stress disorder (PTSD) is a complex mental health condition that often arises in response to experiencing or witnessing a deeply distressing event. The symptoms associated with PTSD can manifest in various ways, including flashbacks, nightmares, intense anxiety, and intrusive thoughts about the traumatic event. These symptoms can significantly disrupt an individual's life, making it challenging to carry out daily activities and maintain overall wellbeing.

## POST-TRAUMATIC GROWTH

The idea that "what doesn't kill you makes you stronger" is widely embraced, echoing a cultural belief in post-traumatic growth (PTG), famously reflected in the lyrics of Kelly Clarkson. This narrative offers hope and optimism in the face of life's challenges and is a fundamental part of the positive health approach.

PTG is a realisation that there is a silver lining in traumatic life events. PTG encompasses five key aspects, which the majority of people experience at some point post-trauma:

- **New possibilities**: Recognising fresh paths and opportunities after trauma, leading to personal growth and development such as making career changes or becoming interested in new hobbies.
- **Relating to others**: Deepening connections with empathy and support from those who have experienced similar challenges, fostering a sense of belonging and a desire to help others.

- **Personal strength**: Acknowledging and building inner resilience, courage, and self-efficacy in overcoming adversity, instilling confidence to face future challenges.
- **Spiritual change**: Reevaluating beliefs to find meaning and purpose amidst suffering, fostering a deeper connection to spirituality or existential understanding.
- **Appreciation of life**: Increased awareness and gratitude for life's beauty and simple pleasures, fostering mindfulness and finding meaning in everyday experiences.

The literature indicates that experiencing PTG does not necessarily alleviate distress or increase happiness; significant growth often accompanies substantial subjective distress (Tedeschi et al., 1998). Also, maintaining growth may require periodic cognitive reminders of loss, ensuring that gains remain a focal point. The objective of PTG is not to fully restore the pre-trauma state of mind, but to enrich individuals' lives, imbuing them with a more significant sense of purpose and fulfilment. As such, PTG contributes to a more meaningful and rewarding existence beyond the adversity endured. Also, given that majority of people experience PTG post-trauma, the process is a natural way of adjustment.

---

### BENEFIT FINDING AND REMINDING

#### (Adapted from King & Miner, 2000; Tennen & Affleck, 2005)

This tool may be helpful to anyone experiencing a traumatic or adverse event, alternatively anyone experiencing chronic illness, alcoholism, or ongoing pain. Reflect on an adverse, traumatic life event or chronic illness you've experienced. Consider the circumstances associated with this event. Now, shift your focus to the positive aspects of this experience. Take a piece of paper and, for the next 20 minutes, write down the following:

- How has this experience benefited you as a person?
- How has this event made you better equipped to cope with challenges in the future?

Don't worry about your spelling or grammar. Nobody is going to read this apart from you. So, let go and explore deeply as you write about the benefits of the challenging experience.

---

It is important to note that empirical evidence supporting PTG is growing but limited. Studies reveal small or insignificant correlations between perceived and actual growth (e.g. Boals et al., 2019), meaning that just because an individual thinks they have grown as a person doesn't mean they have experienced an objectively positive change in their lives. Challenges in assessing growth include participants' memory biases, social desirability pressures, and motivation to perceive growth where it may not actually exist. Therefore, while the idea of adversity leading to growth is compelling, it is crucial to exercise caution and not assume its universality. At the same time, in some cases perceived PTG is enough to motivate people to action and help them live a good life post-trauma; as such, its impact should not be disregarded. More importantly, it is important not to aim to experience PTG. Instead, we can explore a variety of ways to perceive our trauma that helps us heal. PTG could be an outcome of this process.

## CORPOREAL POST-TRAUMATIC GROWTH

Over the last decade a concept of corporeal PTG was introduced, which refers to the transformative changes that take place within an individual's physical being following a traumatic event that change their relationship with the body, such as cancer, burning, or a diagnosis of a chronic disease (Hefferon, 2013). While the concept of PTG has traditionally focused on psychological and emotional aspects, recent research acknowledges the profound impact trauma can have on the body.

One key aspect of corporeal PTG is the development of physical resilience and strength. Trauma often presents physical challenges that push individuals to their limits. Through their own perseverance and adaptation, individuals can emerge from these experiences with increased physical endurance and fortitude. This newfound resilience can manifest in various ways, such as improved muscular strength, enhanced cardiovascular fitness, and a greater capacity to withstand physical stressors.

---

### ONE DOOR CLOSES, ANOTHER DOOR OPENS

**(Adapted from Proyer et al., 2016)**

Every day for the next week, reflect on a time when one door closed in your life (a negative event occurred) and soon after, another door opened (something positive happened as a result of the negative event).

---

Furthermore, corporeal PTG involves the cultivation of a deeper connection with one's body. Trauma can disrupt the mind–body connection, leading to feelings of dissociation or alienation from physical sensations. However, engaging in practices like mindfulness, yoga, or body-based therapies can help individuals re-establish this connection. By tuning into bodily sensations and honouring their physical needs, individuals can develop a profound appreciation for their bodies' resilience and capacity for healing, leading to reduced stress, improved sleep, and enhanced overall wellbeing.

In addition, corporeal PTG may involve adopting healthier lifestyle behaviours as part of the recovery process. Trauma often prompts individuals to reassess their priorities and make conscious choices to prioritise their physical wellbeing. This can include adopting nutritious eating habits, incorporating regular exercise into their routine, and engaging in activities that promote overall wellness. By actively caring for their bodies, individuals not only improve their physical health but also nurture a sense of self-care and self-compassion, acknowledging the importance of their own wellbeing.

Corporeal PTG is not just about physical changes, but also about empowerment. It encompasses a range of positive changes within the physical body following trauma, from building resilience and strength to fostering a deeper mind-body connection and adopting healthier lifestyle behaviours. These transformations contribute to a holistic sense of wellbeing and empowerment in the aftermath of adversity, a concept that is particularly appealing to healthcare professionals and trauma survivors seeking ways to empower themselves or their patients.

## HOW TO EXPERIENCE PTG

Several elements contribute to the promotion of PTG (Henson et al., 2021). Firstly, individuals who engage in sharing negative emotions, engaging in cognitive processing or rumination, and employing positive coping strategies such as positive reappraisal tend to experience higher levels of PTG. This might seem counterintuitive, given that rumination could enhance trauma. However, what is important is an acknowledgement of trauma and the processing of it. Only through this adaptive process will our chances of PTG increase. Additionally, certain personality traits, notably agreeableness, play a role in fostering PTG. These factors need to be considered when working with individuals who have experienced trauma.

Other factors that are important to consider include experiencing multiple sources of trauma, where the trauma is central to one's life events, and can also contribute to PTG. Resilience, as well as engaging in actions that promote personal growth, are key factors in the PTG process. Furthermore, mediators of PTG that indirectly influence its development include seeking social support coping, receiving social support, and maintaining optimism. These factors may not directly cause PTG but can facilitate its emergence.

Interestingly, some studies suggest a positive correlation between PTG and support for aggressive behaviour, implying that the process of growth might be more complex and nuanced than previously understood. Through a systematic exploration of the factors that foster PTG in trauma-exposed professionals, this review aims to provide insights for future research directions. Moreover, it seeks to inform the development of new methods for prevention and intervention tailored specifically for first responders, ultimately enhancing their wellbeing and resilience in the face of trauma.

## LIFESTYLE MEDICINE AND PTSD

Research in this field is still developing. However, initial findings suggest that exercise is a promising treatment for individuals with PTSD (Rosenbaum et al., 2015). Furthermore, considering the increased risk of cardiovascular issues among PTSD patients, in one study a series of lifestyle medicine interventions aimed at improving sleep and exercise was implemented (Kibler et al., 2023).

The results indicated success in achieving the programmes's objectives, although limited information is available regarding PTSD symptoms. Thus, while aiding PTSD patients in reducing non-communicable diseases marks significant progress, exploring the impact of positive psychology and lifestyle medicine interventions in the form of positive health interventions is necessary to assess if a positive focus could aid in maintaining healthy behaviours and decreasing PTSD symptoms.

In summary, PTSD is a complex mental health condition triggered by distressing events that can lead to various symptoms disrupting daily life. At the same time, the concept of PTG can prove useful in positive health, as it guides individuals from experiencing adversity to personal growth, which is one of the components of psychological wellbeing (Ryff & Singer, 1998). PTG encompasses recognising new possibilities, deepening relationships, building personal strength, spiritual re-evaluation, and a greater appreciation for life. While PTG doesn't necessarily alleviate all distress, it can enrich lives and foster a sense of purpose and resilience.

As we have noted, recent attention has been given to corporeal PTG, which acknowledges the body–related changes following trauma. These changes result in a range of psychological adjustments, including increased resilience, a deeper mind–body connection, and healthier lifestyle choices. Factors such as emotional sharing and resilience significantly contribute to PTG, with some studies suggesting a complex relationship with behaviours such as aggression. Understanding these factors is crucial in the context of positive health, as it can guide effective interventions for trauma-exposed individuals, ultimately enhancing their wellbeing and resilience, and equipping them with valuable knowledge.

## EATING DISORDERS

Eating disorders represent significant health challenges that impact both physical wellbeing and mental health. These conditions encompass disturbances in thoughts about food, eating habits, weight, and body shape, manifesting in various eating behaviours. The symptoms associated with eating disorders can profoundly affect an individual's overall health, emotional state, and daily functioning across multiple aspects of life. Common eating disorders include anorexia nervosa, bulimia nervosa, and binge-eating disorder. Anorexia nervosa involves severe restrictions on food intake, often resulting in dangerously low body weight. Bulimia nervosa is characterised by cycles of binge eating followed by purging behaviours to compensate for overeating. Binge-eating disorder entails recurrent episodes of uncontrollable overeating without compensatory behaviours. These disorders not only pose physical health risks but also contribute to emotional distress and impair interpersonal relationships, highlighting the importance of timely intervention and comprehensive treatment approaches.

While much of the existing research on disordered eating tends to concentrate on identifying risk factors, the positive health approach delves into the positive psychological dimensions of this issue. Regrettably, the exploration of positive psychology within the field of eating disorders remains limited, with a predominant emphasis on prevention rather than treatment strategies. Consequently, there is a lack of comprehensive information in this area. The emerging focus on positive body image predominantly centres around adolescents, further narrowing the scope of available research. Expanding this line of enquiry to encompass a broader range of age groups and exploring the potential benefits of positive psychology in both prevention and treatment contexts could offer valuable insights into enhancing the overall wellbeing of individuals affected by eating disorders.

In comparison to the general population, individuals with eating disorders often exhibit lower levels of emotional, psychological, and social wellbeing (de Vos et al., 2018). For instance, while approximately 10% of the general population experiences languishing, over a quarter of individuals with eating disorders report similar wellbeing outcomes. However, intriguingly, a notable percentage of individuals with eating disorders still report flourishing, albeit at an overall lower rate compared to the general population (13%). When examining specific eating disorder conditions, only 9% of individuals with anorexia nervosa and a quarter of those with binge-eating disorder reported flourishing. This suggests that while psychological flourishing is achievable for many individuals with eating disorders. Learning about what they do differently and how flourishing helps them cope with their condition is an interesting area that should be explored in the future.

**BODY GRATITUDE INDUCTION**

**(Dunaev et al., 2018)**

Take a moment to reflect on aspects of your body that you appreciate. This could include various elements such as your health, physical appearance, or the functionality of your body. Aim to identify at least three things, and spend a minute deeply considering them, visualising each one of them in your mind.

Furthermore, the finding that a higher proportion of individuals with eating disorders who binge eat (25%) also report higher psychological flourishing than the general population (approx. 15–17%) raises questions about the nature of overeating behaviour. As such, we need to consider whether overeating could be linked not only to pathological behaviours but also to excessive pursuit of pleasure in food and eating. This complexity of eating disorders needs to be explored in future research to understand the psychological dynamics at play and better and inform more targeted positive health interventions. Consequently, the issue may lie not in overeating per se but in regulating the target of pleasure-seeking behaviour.

### SELF ESTEEM AND EATING DISORDERS

Self-esteem, defined as an individual's perception of self-worth (Rosenberg, 1965), plays a crucial role in understanding disordered eating patterns. Research indicates that low self-esteem is strongly linked to the development and perpetuation of eating disorders and disordered eating behaviours in both men and women. Individuals with these conditions tend to have lower self-esteem compared to healthy individuals and those with other clinical disorders. Conversely, there is evidence suggesting that high self-esteem may act as a protective factor against disordered eating (e.g. Brechan & Kvalem, 2015).

Efforts to prevent and treat disordered eating have started incorporating positive psychology frameworks, focusing on enhancing self-esteem. The rationale for doing it is that by nurturing adolescents' inherent strengths, such as perseverance and kindness, it is believed that overall self-esteem can be boosted, potentially preventing the onset of eating pathology (Gouig, 2006). Weight maintenance programmes showed that strengths of self-regulation, perseverance, love of learning, love of beauty or humour can be particularly beneficial (Pizetta et al., 2022). Programmes aimed at increasing self-esteem have shown promising results in improving eating behaviours and reducing weight and shape concerns among children and adolescents.

Moreover, there is speculation that improving self-esteem could enhance therapeutic outcomes in eating disorder treatment. However, empirical research on self-esteem as a protective factor against disordered eating is still limited, indicating a need for further investigation in this area.

## POSITIVE BODY IMAGE

Exploration of positive body image is a related field to the pathologies of eating disorders. Positive body image encompasses various aspects, such as appreciating one's body, being responsive to needs, and effectively managing threats to body image (Burychka et al., 2021). Having a positive body image can shield individuals from adverse outcomes by directly improving adaptive behaviours and wellbeing, avoiding harmful influences, and navigating detrimental messages. Body image flexibility, which refers to our ability to experience thoughts and feelings about our body without the need to change anything about it (Linardon et al., 2021), is an essential aspect of positive body image. It involves skilfully handling distressing body experiences with openness and non-judgment. Body image flexibility is good for our psyche. It is associated with a reduced risk of eating disorders, body dissatisfaction, and internalised weight bias, along with promoting adaptive eating behaviours and body appreciation. Thus, as part of positive health practice it is essential to consider positive body image.

Numerous weight-loss enterprises focus heavily on exploiting body dissatisfaction as a primary motivator for their programmes. However, research findings suggest a contrasting approach: fostering body satisfaction and positive body image, irrespective of weight and body mass index (BMI), proves more advantageous for weight maintenance. Consequently, messages such as "Are you dissatisfied with your body? Then start a weight-loss programmes" could potentially inflict harm.

---

### SELF-COMPASSIONATE EATING

#### (Adapted from Mantzios & Wilson, 2015)

Each day, allocate 10 minutes to journaling about each aspect of self-compassion – mindfulness, common humanity, and self-kindness – within the framework of healthy eating.
  Mindfulness:
  Reflect on the sensory experience of your food today:

- How does your food look? Describe its colours, textures, and presentation.
- How does your food smell? Identify any aromas and their impact on your appetite.
- How does your food feel? Notice its temperature, texture, and sensations as you eat.

Common Humanity:
  Consider the importance of healthy eating for yourself and others:

- Why is it important for you to eat well? Reflect on how nourishing your body supports your overall wellbeing.
- How does your eating well contribute to the wellbeing of others? Acknowledge the ripple effect of your choices on your loved ones and community.

Self-Kindness:
  Recognise acts of kindness towards yourself through your food choices:

- How are you being kind to yourself by eating this food? Focus on the nourishment and enjoyment it brings you.
- How does your food choice align with your values and self-care goals? Celebrate your efforts to prioritise your health and happiness.

For example, a longitudinal study spanning a decade focusing on overweight adolescent girls revealed that those who maintained satisfaction with their bodies despite being overweight exhibited a greater propensity for effective weight management and sustained a healthy weight trajectory over the years (Loth et al., 2015). This study highlighted the critical importance of nurturing positive body perceptions and challenging the prevailing narrative that equates thinness with happiness and success in weight management endeavours as part of positive health lifestyle changes.

A range of interventions that tapped into the psychology of losing weight and compassion towards body have been developed. For example, a body gratitude activity has increased individuals' intention to exercise and the best possible body activity enhanced their intention to lose weight (Dennis & Ogden, 2023). Thus, it illustrated that positive approaches to a healthy body can prove beneficial.

---

### BEST POSSIBLE BODY

#### (Adapted from Dennis & Ogden, 2023)

To contemplate your "best possible self in terms of aspects of your body", envision yourself having achieved all your body-related goals in the future. Picture this as the culmination of your dreams, where you've reached your body's full potential. This encompasses various elements such as health, physical appearance, and body functionality. Now, jot down a summary of your thoughts and emotions associated with the best possible body I the future. Furthermore, explore the pathways you took to get you there.

---

### SUMMARY

Eating disorders present significant challenges to physical and mental health, encompassing disruptions in eating habits, body image, and weight management. Common disorders like anorexia nervosa, bulimia nervosa, and binge–eating disorder not only jeopardise physical wellbeing but also impact emotional states and daily functioning. While research predominantly focuses on risk factors, exploring positive psychological aspects is important to consider in the context of positive health.

## SCHIZOPHRENIA

More than half of individuals under psychiatric care are diagnosed with schizophrenia, a complex mental illness fraught with stigma. Coping with schizophrenia presents significant challenges for both patients and their families. Schizophrenia is a complex behavioural and cognitive syndrome, severely impacting individual functioning and influencing patient's immediate social environment. Its clinical presentation varies, typically encompassing symptoms such as hallucinations and delusions, emotional blunting, social withdrawal), and cognitive impairment (including inattention and executive dysfunction). Not only must they grapple with the stigma surrounding their condition, but they also contend with a spectrum of symptoms that span the breadth of schizophrenia.

Research involving schizophrenia patients indicates that their baseline quality of life and subjective wellbeing can predict symptom remission and adherence to medication. Consequently, enhancing patients' quality of life, wellbeing, and overall happiness can play a crucial role in preventing relapse and helping them with coping more effectively with disease. Thus, prioritising the wellbeing and recovery of these individuals has become paramount as the multifaceted nature of the illness amplifies the difficulties patients face.

Let us explore some of the positive health topics and activities that have already been used with people diagnosed with schizophrenia.

### WELLBEING

Past research indicated lower levels of psychological flourishing in patients with schizophrenia, in that positive symptoms of schizophrenia exhibit a negative correlation with flourishing, while negative symptoms are predictive of languishing (Pina et al., 2021). Positive symptoms, including hallucinations and delusions, may hinder individuals from experiencing happiness and finding meaning in life. These symptoms not only present challenges to the individual's mental health but also impede their ability to engage fully in daily activities and pursue fulfilling experiences. Consequently, addressing these symptoms is crucial for promoting overall wellbeing and enhancing the quality of life for individuals living with schizophrenia.

A longitudinal study with patients diagnosed with schizophrenia found that, although a higher percentage of them languished (19.3%) compared to the general population, over half reported moderate wellbeing (52.5%), and almost a third (28.2%) flourished psychologically while coping with their schizophrenia (Chan et al., 2018). This research demonstrates that it is possible to flourish despite having Schizophrenia Spectrum Disorder. Additionally, six months later, those who reported higher levels of clinical recovery – meaning their symptoms had reduced to a level that allowed them to reclaim autonomy and function in daily life – also reported higher levels of wellbeing. The study offers hope for anyone experiencing this challenging disorder.

A comprehensive review of positive health interventions has brought to light a promising future for mental healthcare, revealing significant improvements in patients' wellbeing. While the effectiveness of these interventions in reducing negative symptoms of schizophrenia varied (Pina et al., 2021), the research indicated that specific wellbeing enhancements persisted for up to three months post-intervention. These enhancements, including life satisfaction, hope, resilience, and self-esteem, are not just temporary boosts but psychological resources that can equip individuals with schizophrenia for a more fulfilling life. Additionally, some studies reported decreases in anhedonia (the inability to experience pleasure) and apathy (lack of interest). However, one study found no changes in emotional experiences among participants. Interventions such as mental fitness training, meditation practices, and integrating positive psychology activities like gratitude or savouring into daily routines demonstrated promising results. Therefore, positive health initiatives serve as a solid foundation for enhancing the lives of individuals with schizophrenia, offering a glimmer of hope and optimism for the future of mental healthcare.

## STIGMA

In recent times, a variety of positive psychology interventions have emerged for individuals with schizophrenia, yielding mixed results.

One such intervention is Positive Psychology Expressive Writing (PPEW), tailored to combat the stigma associated with schizophrenia, particularly among female patients (Tang et al., 2023). Participants engaged in a six-week pre-recorded training to address topics like confronting trauma, focusing on its silver linings, exploring positivity, cultivating gratitude, embracing happiness, and revitalising hope. Following each session, participants were prompted to articulate their thoughts through writing.

The outcomes revealed a reduction in stigma among patients and a newfound sense of hope for the future. Additionally, the intervention facilitated the expression of thoughts and encouraged reframing them in a positive light, thereby aiding in the more effective management of schizophrenia symptoms. Importantly, as individuals with schizophrenia often struggle to trust others and express their emotions, this activity provided a safe platform for expression without fear of judgement.

The skills cultivated through this intervention were diverse, encompassing attentional strategies, fostering positive relationships, enhancing verbal communication, and nurturing trust and hope.

## POSITIVE PSYCHOTHERAPY

Researchers investigating interventions for individuals with schizophrenia advocate for the integration of positive psychotherapy into clinical practice (Sawicka & Żochowska, 2019). They contend that positive psychotherapy offers a multitude of advantages for schizophrenic patients, including enhancing positive experiences, cultivating positive emotions, improving wellbeing, and facilitating the use of their strengths. By focusing on these aspects, positive psychotherapy holds promise for improving the overall wellbeing and functioning of individuals grappling with schizophrenia. Its emphasis on leveraging inherent strengths and fostering positivity aligns with the holistic approach necessary for effective treatment in this population. Thus, practitioners are encouraged to consider positive psychotherapy as a valuable addition to their therapeutic toolkit for addressing the complex needs of schizophrenic patients. This could be especially beneficial for newly diagnosed patients (Halverson et al., 2021).

Positive experiences are a significant challenge for individuals with schizophrenia due to the limitations imposed by the illness.

Thus, interventions that promote positive emotions in this population are crucial. For instance, "Positive Living", a group psychotherapy programme aimed at enhancing hope, enjoyment, satisfaction, and self-esteem among individuals with schizophrenia (Meyer et al., 2012). This ten-session programme resulted in notable improvements in hope, wellbeing, and the ability to enjoy life, along with reduced psychotic and depressive symptoms. Participants also reported improved interpersonal relationships and decreased focus on psychotic experiences, with benefits sustained three months post-therapy.

Character strengths are beneficial in enhancing positive experiences. Therapeutic efforts have traditionally focused on cultivating strengths such as kindness, gratitude, and forgiveness. In the context of interventions tailored for schizophrenic patients, it is proposed that focusing on kindness as a primary strength may be particularly beneficial for patients (Johnson et al., 2009). Kindness is a powerful motivator for offering unconditional and voluntary assistance, providing a valuable framework for promoting positive experiences and wellbeing in this population. However, we hope that future research will explore more strengths beneficial for schizophrenic patients to use.

## LIFESTYLE MEDICINE AND SCHIZOPHRENIA

For decades, individuals diagnosed with schizophrenia have been noted for their suboptimal lifestyle habits. Research indicates their diet tends to be higher in fat and lower in fibre compared to the general population, with reduced physical activity levels, although not necessarily leading to obesity. Additionally, they exhibit heavy smoking habits but consume less alcohol (Brown et al., 1999). Recent studies have revealed correlations between patients' lifestyles and the severity of their schizophrenia, emphasising the pressing need for lifestyle medicine interventions (Kalinowska et al., 2021). Among the recommended interventions for schizophrenia patients is lifestyle coaching (Kanofsky et al., 2022). Considering the positive outcomes of positive psychology interventions, integrating them with lifestyle medicine interventions as positive health approaches could offer significant benefits for this population. Further research is warranted to explore this connection in greater depth.

## SUMMARY

Individuals diagnosed with schizophrenia often face significant challenges, with the illness affecting both their personal wellbeing and social interactions. Symptoms like hallucinations, delusions, emotional blunting, and cognitive impairment contribute to the complexity of the condition. Additionally, stigma further complicates the lives of those affected. However, research suggests that interventions focusing on positive health and wellbeing can have substantial benefits for individuals with schizophrenia. These interventions, including positive psychology techniques like expressive writing and positive psychotherapy, aim to improve quality of life, foster resilience, and enhance positive emotions. Positive psychotherapy, in particular, emphasises leveraging individuals' strengths and promoting positivity to address the multifaceted challenges of schizophrenia. Initiatives like "Positive Living" have shown promising results in enhancing hope, satisfaction, and self-esteem among schizophrenic patients while also reducing psychotic and depressive symptoms. Thus, integrating positive interventions into clinical practice holds significant promise for improving the lives of individuals with schizophrenia, offering hope for enhanced wellbeing and recovery.

## POSITIVE HEALTH IN MENTAL DISORDER

In this chapter, we explored limited mental health issues and highlighted existing research in positive health. Our main objective was to inspire mental health professionals to incorporate positive health books and approaches into their patients' care. Evidence is increasingly showing the benefits of applying positive psychology and lifestyle medicine interventions with patients who have mental disorders. We hope this chapter serves as a starting point for exploring other conditions your patients may have and discovering ways to use positive health to help them cope with symptoms or flourish despite their disorder. After all, everyone deserves the right to live a good life, regardless of their condition.

# REFERENCES

Biskas, M., Cheung, W. Y., Juhl, J., Sedikides, C., Wildschut, T., & Hepper, E. (2019). A prologue to nostalgia: Savouring creates nostalgic memories that foster optimism. *Cognition & Emotion*, *33*(3), 417–427. https://doi.org/10.1080/02699931.2018.1458705

Boals, A., Bedford, L.A., & Callahan, J.L. (2019). Perceptions of change after a trauma and perceived posttraumatic growth: A prospective examination. *Behavioral Science* (Basel), *9*(1), 10. https://doi.org/10.3390/bs9010010

Brechan, I., & Kvalem, I. L. (2015). Relationship between body dissatisfaction and disordered eating: Mediating role of self-esteem and depression. *Eating Behaviors*, *17*, 49–58. https://doi.org/10.1016/j.eatbeh.2014.12.008

Brown, L., Ospina, J. P., Celano, C. M., Huffman, J.C. (2019). The effects of positive psychological interventions on medical patients' anxiety: A meta-analysis. *Psychosomatic Medicine*, *81*(7), 595–602. doi: 10.1097/PSY.0000000000000722

Brown, S., Birtwistle, J., Roe, L., & Thompson, C. (1999). The unhealthy lifestyle of people with schizophrenia. *Psychological Medicine*, *29*(3), 697–701. https://doi.org/10.1017/s0033291798008186

Burychka, D., Miragall, M., Baños, R. M. (2021). Towards a comprehensive understanding of body image: Integrating positive body image, embodiment and self-compassion. *Psychologica Belgica*, *61*(1), 248–261. https://doi.org/10.5334/pb.1057

Carr, A., Finneran, L., Boyd, C., Shirey, C., Canning, C., Stafford, O., … Burke, T. (2024). The evidence-base for positive psychology interventions: a mega-analysis of meta-analyses. *The Journal of Positive Psychology*, *19*(2), 191–205. https://doi.org/10.1080/17439760.2023.2168564

Carr, A., Cullen, K., Keeney, C., Canning, C., Mooney, O., Chinseallaigh, E., & O'Dowd, A. (2021). Effectiveness of positive psychology interventions: A systematic review and meta-analysis. *The Journal of Positive Psychology*, *16*(6), 749–769. https://doi.org/10.1080/17439760.2020.1818807

Chan, R. C. H., Mak, W. W. S., Chio, F. H. N., & Tong, A. C. Y. (2018). Flourishing with psychosis: A prospective examination on the interactions between clinical, functional, and personal recovery processes on well-being among individuals with schizophrenia spectrum disorders. *Schizophrenia Bulletin*, 44(4), 778–786. https://doi.org/10.1093/schbul/sbx120

Corrigan, P. W., & Phelan, S. M. (2004). Social support and recovery in people with serious mental illnesses. *Community Mental Health Journal*, *40*(6), 513–523. https://doi.org/10.1007/s10597-004-6125-5

Daley, A. (2008). Exercise and depression: A review of reviews. *Journal of Clinical Psychology in Medical Settings*, *15*(2), 140–147. https://doi.org/10.1007/s10880-008-9105-z

Dein, S. (2006). Religion, spirituality and depression: Implications for research and treatment. *Primary Care & Community Psychiatry*, *11*(2), 67–72. https:// doi.org/10.1185/135525706X121110

de Vos, J. A., Radstaak, M., Bohlmeijer, E. T., & Westerhof, G. J. (2018). Having an eating disorder and still being able to flourish? Examination of pathological symptoms and well-being as two continua of mental health in a clinical sample. *Frontiers in Psychology*, *9*, 2145. https://doi.org/10.3389/ fpsyg.2018.02145

Dennis, A., & Ogden, J. (2023).The effect of body-focused positive psychology interventions on behavioural intentions, body esteem, and body compassion. *International Journal of Applied Positive Psychology*. https://doi. org/10.1007/s41042-023-00134-1

Dunaev, J., Markey, C. H., & Brochu, P. M. (2018). An attitude of gratitude: The effects of body-focused gratitude on weight bias internalization and body image. *Body Image*, *25*, 9–13. https://doi.org/10.1016/j.bodyim.2018. 01.006

Fuller-Thomson, E., Agbeyaka, S., LaFond, D. M., & Bern-Klug, M. (2016). Flourishing after depression: Factors associated with achieving complete mental health among those with a history of depression. *Psychiatry Research*, *242*, 111–120. https://doi.org/10.1016/j.psychres.2016.04.041

Gilmour, H. (2014). Positive mental health and mental illness. *Health Reports*, *25*(9), 3–9.

Gouig, S. (2006). Preventing eating disorders in young adolescents using positive psychology (Order No. AAI3215394). Available from PsycINFO (621574136; 2006-99020-99344).

Halverson, T. F., Meyer-Kalos, P. S., Perkins, D. O., Gaylord, S. A., Palsson, O. S., Nye, L., Algoe, S. B., Grewen, K., & Penn, D. L. (2021). Enhancing stress reactivity and wellbeing in early schizophrenia: A randomized controlled trial of Integrated Coping Awareness Therapy (I-CAT). *Schizophrenia Research*, *235*, 91–101. https://doi.org/10.1016/j.schres.2021.07.022

Hefferon, K. (2013). *Positive psychology and body: The somatopsychic side to flourishing*. Open University Press.

Henson, C., Truchot, D., & Canevello, A. (2021). What promotes post traumatic growth? A systematic review. *European Journal of Trauma & Dissociation*, *5*(4), 100195. https://doi.org/10.1016/j.ejtd.2020.100195

Hoffman, R., Gimenez Hinkle, M., & Kress, V. W. (2010). Letter writing as an intervention in family therapy with adolescents who engage in nonsuicidal self-injury. *The Family Journal*, *18*(1), 24–30. https://doi. org/10.1177/1066480709355039

Johnson, D. P., Penn, D. L., Fredrickson, B. L., Meyer, P. S., Kring, A. M., & Brantley, M. (2009). Loving: Kindness meditation on enhance recovery from negative symptoms of schizophrenia. *Journal of Clinical Psychology*, *65*, 499–509.

Kalinowska, S., Kłoda, K., Safranow, K., Misiak, B., Cyran, A., & Samochowiec, J. (2021). The association between lifestyle choices and schizophrenia symptoms. *Journal of Clinical Medicine*, *10*(1), 165. https://doi.org/10.3390/jcm10010165

Kanofsky, J. D., Viswanathan, S., & Wylie-Rosett, J. (2022). Lifestyle coaching may be an effective treatment for schizophrenia. *American Journal of Lifestyle Medicine*, *18*(2), 156–161. https://doi.org/10.1177/15598276221142307

Kibler, J., Ma, M., Hrzich, J., & Choe, J. (2023). Pilot findings indicate a cognitive behavioral healthy lifestyle intervention for PTSD improves sleep and physical activity. *Brain Sciences*, *13*(11), 1565. https://doi.org/10.3390/brainsci13111565

King, L. A., & Miner, K. N. (2000). Writing about the perceived benefits of traumatic events: Implications for physical health. *Personality and Social Psychology Bulletin*, *26*(2), 220–230. https://doi.org/10.1177/0146167200264008

Linardon, J., Anderson, C., Messer, M., Rodgers, R. F., & Fuller-Tyszkiewicz, M. (2021). Body image flexibility and its correlates: A meta-analysis. *Body Image*, *37*, 188–203. https://doi.org/10.1016/j.bodyim.2021.02.005

Lopez, S. J., Snyder, C. R., Magyar-Moe, J. L., Edwards, L. M., Pedrotti, J. T., Janowski, K., Turner, J. L., & Pressgrove, C. (2004). Strategies for accentuating hope. In P. A. Linley & S. Joseph (Eds.), *Positive psychology in practice* (pp. 388–404). John Wiley. https://doi.org/10.1002/9780470939338.ch24

Loth, K. A., Watts, A. W., van den Berg, P., & Neumark-Sztainer, D. (2015). Does body satisfaction help or harm overweight teens? A 10-year longitudinal study of the relationship between body satisfaction and body mass index. *Journal of Adolescent Health* (official publication of the Society for Adolescent Medicine), *57*(5), 559–561. https://doi.org/10.1016/j.jadohealth.2015.07.008

Mantzios, M., & Wilson, J.C. (2015). Mindfulness, Eating Behaviours, and Obesity: A Review and Reflection on Current Findings. *Current Obesity Reports*, *4*, 141–146. https://doi.org/10.1007/s13679-014-0131-x

Meyer, P. S., Johnson, D. P., Parks, A., Iwansky, C., & Penn, D. L. (2012). Positive living: A pilot study pf group positive psychotherapy for people with schizophrenia. *Journal of Positive Psychology*, *7*, 239–248.

Pina, I., Braga, C. de M., de Oliveira, T. lio F. R., de Santana, C. N., Marques, R. C., & Machado, L. (2021). Positive psychology interventions to improve wellbeing and symptoms in people on the schizophrenia spectrum: A systematic review and meta-analysis. *Brazilian Journal of Psychiatry / Revista Brasileira de Psiquiatria*, *43*(4), 430–437. https://doi.org/10.1590/1516-4446-2020-1164

Piran, N., Teall, T. L., & Counsell, A. (2020). The experience of embodiment scale: Development and psychometric evaluation. *Body Image*, *34*, 117–134. https://doi.org/10.1016/j.bodyim.2020.05.007

Pizetta, A., Mello, L.T.N., & Andretta, I. (2022). Character strengths in weight maintenance: perceptions after a weight loss programmes. *Psicologia Argumento*, *40*(111). https://doi.org/10.7213/psicolargum.40.111.AO08

Proyer, R. T., Gander, F., & Tandler, N. (2016). Strength-based interventions. *Gifted Education International*, *33*(2). https://doi.org/10.1177/0261429416640334

Rosenbaum, S., Tiedemann, A., Berle, D., Ward, P. B., & Zachary, S. (2015). Exercise as a novel treatment option to address cardiometabolic dysfunction associated with PTSD. *Metabolism: Clinical and Experimental*, *64*(5), e5–e6. https://doi.org/10.1016/j.metabol.2015.01.016h

Rosenberg, M. (1965). *Society and the adolescent self-image*. Princeton University Press. https://doi.org/10.1515/9781400876136

Ryff, C. D., & Singer, B. (1998). The contours of positive human health. *Psychological Inquiry*, *9*(1), 1–28. https://doi.org/10.1207/s15327965pli0901_1

Sawicka, M., & Żochowska, A. (2018). Positive interventions in the therapy of schizophrenia patients. *Current Problems of Psychiatry*, *19*(4), 239–247. https://doi.org/10.2478/cpp-2018-0018

Schotanus-Dijkstra, M., Ten Have, M., Lamers, S. M. A., de Graaf, R., & Bohlmeijer, E. T. (2017). The longitudinal relationship between flourishing mental health and incident mood, anxiety and substance use disorders. *European Journal of Public Health*, *27*(3), 563–568. doi: 10.1093/eurpub/ckw202

Steger, M. F., Shim, Y., Barenz, J., & Shin, J. Y. (2014). Through the windows of the soul: A pilot study using photography to enhance meaning in life. *Journal of Contextual Behavioral Science*, *3*(1), 27–30. https://doi.org/10.1016/j.jcbs.2013.11.002

Tang, M.-W., Cheng, Y., Zhang, Y.-H., & Liu, S.-J. (2023). Effect of a positive psychology expressive writing on stigma, hope, coping style, and quality of life in hospitalized female patients with schizophrenia: A randomized, controlled trial. *Perspectives in Psychiatric Care*, 1–12. https://doi.org/10.1155/2023/1577352

Tedeschi, R. G., Park, C. L., & Calhoun, L. G. (Eds.) (1998). *Posttraumatic growth: Positive changes in the aftermath of crisis*. Lawrence Erlbaum.

Tennen, H., & Affleck, G. (2005). Benefit-finding and benefit-reminding. In C. R. Snyder & S. J. Lopez (Eds.), *Handbook of positive psychology* (pp. 584–597). Oxford University Press.

Voica, S. A., Kling, J., Frisén, A., & Piran, N. (2021). Disordered eating through the lens of positive psychology: The role of embodiment, self-esteem and identity coherence. *Body Image*, *39*, 103–113. https://doi.org/10.1016/j.bodyim.2021.06.006

Wellenzohn, S., Proyer, R. T., & Ruch, W. (2016). How do positive psychology interventions work? A short-term placebo-controlled humor-based study on the role of the time focus. *Personality and Individual Differences*, *96*, 1–6. https://doi.org/10.1016/j.paid.2016.02.056

Westerhof, G. J., & Keyes, C. L. (2010). Mental illness and mental health: The two continua model across the lifespan. *Journal of Adult Development, 17*(2), 110–119. https://doi.org/10.1007/s10804-009-9082-y

Wong, V. W. H., Ho, F. Y. Y., Shi, N., Sarris, J., Chung, K., & Yeung, W. (2021). Lifestyle medicine for depression: A meta-analysis of randomized controlled trials. *Journal of Affective Disorders, 284*, 203–216. https://doi.org/10.1016/j.jad.2021.02.012

Wong, V. W. H., Ho, F. Y. Y., Shi, N., Sarris, J., Ng, C. H., & Tam, O. K. Y. (2022). Lifestyle medicine for anxiety symptoms: A meta-analysis of randomized controlled trials. *Journal of Affective Disorders, 310*, 354–368. https://doi.org/10.1016/j.jad.2022.04.151

Worthington, E. L., Kurusu, T. A., Collins, W., Berry, J. W., Ripley, J. S., & Baier, S. N. (2000). Forgiving usually takes time: A lesson learned by studying interventions to promote forgiveness. *Journal of Psychology and Theology, 28*(1), 3–20. https://doi.org/10.1177/009164710002800101

# 4

# POSITIVE PHYSICAL HEALTH

Lifestyle medicine is a crucial approach that harnesses evidence-based lifestyle and therapeutic interventions to not just manage, but also prevent and reverse non–communicable diseases (NCDs). These encompass a wide range of health conditions, from cardiovascular disease (CVD) and lung disease (such as chronic obstructive pulmonary disease and asthma), to Type 2 diabetes, metabolic syndrome, certain cancers, mental health issues, and suicide (WHO, 2021).

---

**WORLD HEALTH ORGANISATION (WHO) STATISTICS ON NONCOMMUNICABLE DISEASES (NCDs)**

NCDs kill 41 million people each year, equivalent to 74% of all deaths globally.

Each year, 17 million people die from a NCD before age 70; 86% of these premature deaths occur in low- and middle-income countries.

Of all NCD deaths, 77% are in low- and middle-income countries.

Cardiovascular diseases account for most NCD deaths, or 17.9 million people annually, followed by cancers (9.3 million), chronic respiratory diseases (4.1 million), and diabetes (2.0 million including kidney disease deaths caused by diabetes).

---

DOI: 10.4324/9781003457169-4

These four groups of diseases account for over 80% of all premature NCD deaths.

Tobacco use, physical inactivity, the harmful use of alcohol, unhealthy diets and air pollution all increase the risk of dying from an NCD.

Source: https://www.who.int/news-room/fact-sheets/detail/noncommunicable-diseases

The six pillars of lifestyle medicine are (1) stress management techniques and behaviours; (2) a predominantly whole food, plant-based diet; (3) daily physical activity; (4) adequate sleep; (5) avoiding risky substances, particularly tobacco and alcohol; and (6) social engagement (fostering relationships with others) (ACLM, 2022). Our research indicates that lifestyle–medicine–based interventions, which promote adequate sleep, healthy eating, stress management, and daily physical activity, combined with positive psychology practices – such as adopting a growth mindset and cultivating gratitude and optimism – have a synergistic, beneficial impact on overall health (Burke & Dunne, 2022). Additionally, integrating lifestyle medicine and positive psychology practices with Health Psychology approaches can help individuals develop sustainable positive lifestyle habits, enabling them to thrive (Lianov & Burke, 2023).

In this chapter, we will delve into the concept of positive physical health and present research and real-life examples of its application to enhance overall health. Before we explore how a healthy lifestyle, aligned with the six pillars, can prevent or manage NCDs, it's important to understand the biological mechanisms and interfaces that underpin health. A key principle is homeostasis, the balance that all systems require. Disruption of this balance can lead to social inequality, environmental catastrophe (climate change), and disease (both mental and physical). Lifestyle medicine plays a crucial role in maintaining this balance.

## BRAIN (MIND)–BODY CONNECTIONS AND THE PHYSICAL ENVIRONMENT

Understanding the intricate connection between the brain, mind, body and the physical environment is crucial for fostering positive health. The analogy of the human body as a doughnut, familiar to many undergraduate students, depicts the intricate relationship between our physiology and the surrounding environment. Our skin is the outer layer of the doughnut, while the central ring represents the linings of our gastrointestinal tract and lungs. By embracing this perspective, we empower ourselves to make informed choices that support our wellbeing and positive health, and foster harmony between ourselves and our environment.

We, as human beings, are constantly exposed to trillions of molecules in the air we breathe, the food we eat, and the materials we touch daily. The endothelial and epithelial layers of our skin, the cell lining of our gastrointestinal tract, and the alveolar cells of our lungs act as barriers to the external environment, but they are also permeable, allowing environmental molecules to pass through. This is necessary for us to digest and absorb nutrients from food in the gut and exchange waste carbon dioxide for oxygen through the lungs. In essence, we are intricately connected to our environment. Therefore, our physical health is not only influenced by our personal choices but also by the state of our environment, the climate, the nature of our food, and the quality of the air we breathe.

Positive health emphasises the importance of maintaining this delicate balance, recognising that our physical wellbeing is deeply intertwined with our surroundings. On this planet, we coexist with a multitude of other living organisms, both large and small. Beyond being obvious sources of food and medicine, the plant life that surrounds us plays a vital role. It produces the oxygen we breathe, a necessity for most life on Earth. Trees also emit volatile organic chemicals (VOCs) such as limonene, pinene, and terpenes, which have been proven to be beneficial for human health. These VOCs can enhance our immune system, improve cognition and mood, and even promote health through activities like "forest bathing" (Hansen et al., 2017). The sheer beauty of nature itself can also have significant health benefits for humans (Bratman et al., 2021).

It has also become increasingly apparent that contact with other mammals (especially domesticated animals) plays a role in training our immune system to become tolerant during early life. Animals can expose young humans to various environmental molecules such as dander, as well as microbial species (bacteria, viruses, yeast, and archaea), all of which can educate and train the immune system not to overreact in later life (Jain, 2020). Many scientists believe that the pursuit of sterility in our homes and workplaces through the use of detergents and antiseptics has contributed to the increasing numbers of humans who develop hyper-reactive immune systems, such as allergies, asthma, and certain autoimmune diseases. This is known as the hygiene hypothesis (Pfefferle et al., 2021).

Over the past few decades, it has become increasingly clear that microbial species (bacteria, viruses, yeast, and archaea) living both inside and outside our bodies are essential for human health. These vast collections of microbial species are grouped into living environments called microbiomes. Humans have microbiomes associated with our skin, reproductive organs, gastrointestinal tract, and lungs (Ursell et al., 2012).

The gut microbiome, a vast population estimated at 40 trillion, is composed of bacteria, viruses, yeast, and archaea. The diversity of these microbiomes is often as distinct as a human fingerprint (Cryan et al., 2019). These organisms, also known as probiotics, play a crucial role in maintaining our health. They promote a functioning immune system, communicate with the nervous system (enteric and autonomic nerves), balance insulin and blood glucose, aid in nutrient absorption, and produce neurotransmitters that help regulate our mood (Grenham et al., 2011).

In positive health, we explore the intricate interplay between the human body, its environment, and microbial communities. By understanding and embracing these holistic dynamics, we pave the way for a comprehensive approach to wellbeing that transcends the mere absence of disease, encompassing physical vitality, mental resilience, and environmental harmony. Through this lens, we embark on a journey to unlock the full potential of positive health, where the synergy between humanity and its surroundings fosters thriving individuals and flourishing communities. Let us now delve into real-life example to illustrate this transformative vision.

### The Johnsons' journey

*Once upon a time in a small suburban neighbourhood lived the Johnson family. Tom and Sarah Johnson were devoted parents to two young children, Emma and Jake. They believed a spotless, germ-free* home was essential for their children's wellbeing, and thus, they meticulously cleaned every surface with powerful detergents and antiseptics daily.

At first, the Johnsons' home was a pristine haven, the scent of cleaning agents providing a reassuring sense of safety. But as time went on, Emma and Jake's health took a turn for the worse. They were plagued by constant colds, allergies, and asthma, leading to a string of doctor visits that offered no solutions. Tom and Sarah were left feeling helpless and confused.

It was during one of these visits, as Sarah was waiting at the doctor's office, that she stumbled upon an article that would change everything. It discussed the hygiene hypothesis and the human microbiome, suggesting that excessive cleanliness could actually weaken the immune system. It also highlighted the health benefits of exposure to environmental microbes and the positive effects of nature, such as the health-promoting volatile organic chemicals (VOCs) released by trees.

Intrigued, Sarah researched further and discovered that contact with animals and exposure to natural environments were crucial in training the immune system during early life. She realised their overly sterile home had deprived Emma and Jake of essential microbial exposure, leading to overactive immune responses.

With this newfound knowledge, the Johnsons embarked on a journey to restore balance. They replaced harsh cleaning agents with gentler, eco-friendly alternatives. They encouraged Emma and Jake to spend more time outdoors, exploring the nearby park and even tending to a small garden. And they welcomed a furry friend, Max, into their home, who not only brought joy but also introduced beneficial microbes.

Gradually, Emma and Jake's health improved. Their frequent illnesses subsided, allergies and asthma symptoms diminished, and they became more energetic and happy. The simple act of reconnecting with nature and allowing their children to experience the world around them made all the difference.

The Johnsons' story reminds us of the balance between cleanliness and natural exposure. By fostering a healthy relationship with the environment and understanding the importance of microbial diversity, they discovered a path to better health and wellbeing. Their once overly sterile home was now filled with laughter, the joy of a playful dog, and the vibrant life of a blooming garden.

## THE BRAIN (MIND)–BODY CONNECTION

In positive health, understanding the intricate relationship between the mind and body is paramount. The brain, a very complex organ, defies full description within the confines of a single chapter. This short section highlights that our brain, and, by default, our mind, is connected to our body and vice versa. This is an obvious statement to make. However, much of science and medicine over the past 300 hundred years has artificially created a duality of body and mind; this is primarily blamed on the French philosopher Rene Descartes, who died in 1650 (Thibaut, 2018). We have developed an ever-greater specialism in science that reduces the workings of the brain and body into silos, which help us to understand the essential workings of these complex biological systems. Our brain, mind, and body represent one integrated system that interfaces constantly with our external (social, physical, ecological) and internal (biological and thinking process) environments.

Furthermore, what we think and perceive can impact our biology; likewise, our environments can impact our thinking processes, perceptions, and biology. Humans exist in an exquisitely beautiful and almost infinitely complex dance with nature. An imbalance in any one of the brain, mind, body, or environment can negatively impact our overall health.

The brain is divided into two hemispheres (left and right) connected by the corpus callosum, associated with different functions, states, and traits. The reality might be more complex, which is beautifully described in a book by scientist and psychiatrist Ian McGilchrist (McGilchrist, 2012). A cross-sectional view of the brain (imagine cutting a cake in half to view the inherent layers) reveals three essential areas: the old brain (reptilian), the limbic brain (old mammals), and the neocortex (new mammals) (Figure 4.1).

## INTEROCEPTION AND EMOTIONS

One essential process for understanding the mind–body connection is interoception, our brain's perception of bodily states transmitted by receptors in our internal organs. Interoception involves how the nervous system anticipates, senses, interprets, integrates, and regulates bodily signals on both unconscious and conscious levels

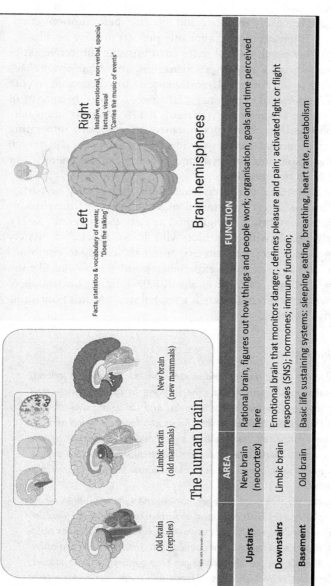

| AREA | | FUNCTION |
|---|---|---|
| **Upstairs** | New brain (neocortex) | Rational brain, figures out how things and people work; organisation, goals and time perceived here |
| **Downstairs** | Limbic brain | Emotional brain that monitors danger; defines pleasure and pain; activated fight or flight responses (SNS); hormones; immune function; |
| **Basement** | Old brain | Basic life sustaining systems: sleeping, eating, breathing, heart rate, metabolism |

*Figure 4.1* The Human brain. The brain is divided into two hemispheres (left and right) that have been associated with different functions. A cross-sectional view of the brain reveals the old reptilian, limbic, and neocortical sections. Each area is associated with (1) sustaining basic life functions (heart beat and breathing), (2) emotional regulation, memory and sensory perception, and (3) logical and rational thinking, respectively. This figure was generated using licensed BioRender software.

(Khalsa et al., 2018). When individuals struggle to detect these signals, they are less likely to notice and regulate their emotions effectively. Thus, interoception significantly impacts positive health.

Emotions are psychological states encompassing subjective experiences, physiological responses, cognitions, and expressive behaviours linked to motivational reorientation. Interoception, a core element of emotional experiences, facilitates adaptive behaviour in response to the environment (Barrett, 2017). Multiple brain networks collaborate to construct instances of emotion, integrating interoceptive information to provide basic affective feelings such as pleasure, displeasure, arousal, and calmness. Consequently, our emotions become embodied.

Research indicates that individuals with anxiety may be particularly skilled at detecting internal organ signals but often misinterpret them, resulting in heightened anxiety (Slotta et al., 2021). Conversely, people with depression who do not experience anxiety may struggle to detect their internal processes, leading to emotional numbness and an inability to experience positive emotions like joy, happiness, or hope (Furman et al., 2013). Training our minds to connect with our internal body is a crucial step towards flourishing and positive health.

### Amahle's story

*Amahle is a single mother and recent economic migrant to Ireland, originally from South Africa. She is living in an under-resourced neighbourhood in the Dublin suburbs, and struggling with chronic stress and fatigue. She works long hours at a low-paying job and has little time for herself. Her children, ages 7 and 5, are often ill, adding to her stress. Maria read about positive health sciences on a local government website and decided to incorporate some of its principles into her life.*

*She started with small changes, introducing a predominantly whole food, plant-based diet. Her local supermarket had regular deals in fresh fruit and vegetables that she used to cook the food of her childhood; it also kept her children connected to their South African heritage. Amahle and her children began eating more fruits, vegetables, and legumes, replacing processed foods, which are often cheaper than healthy foods. Maria also set aside time each evening for a brief walk* with her kids, making physical activity a fun family event. These walks not only improve their physical health but also strengthen their bond as a family and with the local community.

Amahle learned about stress management techniques from a group of other recent African migrants who meet weekly online. She finds it easier to practice these techniques with like-minded people in a group setting rather than alone. She began practising meditation for a few minutes each morning and finds that helps her to regulate her emotions. The group meetings make her feel less lonely and more connected to other people. In an attempt to tackle her fatigue, she introduced sleep hygiene with routines that include reading to her children before bedtime. This helps the whole family to get adequate sleep and establishes a consistent bedtime routine. It is not always perfect but everyone feels a little better during the day these days.

Over time, Amahle has noticed significant improvements in her well-being. Her energy levels are gradually increasing, her children's health has stabilised, and she feels more resilient against stress. Embracing positive health science practices has transformed Amahle's life, providing her and her family with a pathway to better health and happiness.

## POSITIVE EMBODIMENT

Positive embodiment is defined as experiencing comfort and connection with the body, attuned self-care, and bodily agency (Piran, 2016). "Agency" in this context refers to the ability to use the body effectively and confidently in various activities, such as sports, social events, or even walking through a crowded street. It contrasts with disrupted embodiment, characterised by discomfort, self-neglect, and restricted agency (Piran, 2016). Positive embodiment involves feeling at ease in one's body, being attentive and responsive to its needs, and having the ability to use the body effectively and confidently in various activities.

For example, someone experiencing positive embodiment might enjoy physical activities such as yoga or dance, feeling in tune with their body's movements and rhythms. They listen to their body's signals, such as hunger or fatigue, and respond with appropriate self-care practices like eating nourishing foods and getting sufficient rest. This person feels a sense of agency, confidently engaging in activities without fear or discomfort, whether playing a sport, participating in a social event, or simply walking through a crowded street.

In stark contrast, someone experiencing disrupted embodiment might feel disconnected from their body, experiencing it more as a source of discomfort or pain. They may ignore or misinterpret their body's signals, leading to self-neglect, such as skipping meals or pushing through exhaustion without rest. This person might feel restricted in their activities, avoiding physical or social engagements due to a lack of confidence or fear of judgment, thus limiting their ability to fully participate in life. This highlights the significant impact of disrupted embodiment on one's daily life and overall wellbeing.

Positive embodiment fosters a holistic sense of wellbeing and enhances one's overall quality of life. It empowers the body, making it a source of strength and comfort. This state of positive embodiment supports mental and emotional health, enabling individuals to pursue their goals and engage with their environment in meaningful ways. In contrast, disrupted embodiment can hinder one's daily functioning and overall satisfaction, emphasising the crucial role of nurturing a positive relationship with one's body.

Positive embodiment is therefore an amalgamation of a variety of concepts such as intuitive eating (Tylka & Kroon Van Diest, 2013) and positive sexuality (Hefferon, 2013), shifting the focus from treating disorders and problems to offering solutions. Emerging research supports this approach, showing that, for example, overweight adolescents who were satisfied with their bodies rather than critical of them were more likely to maintain a healthy weight a decade later. Exploring positive embodiment in various aspects of lifestyle medicine can significantly enhance both body and mind, making it a formidable task with substantial potential for improving overall wellbeing, or "embodied wellbeing" (Piran et al., 2020).

## STRESS AND THE BRAIN (THE PSYCHO-NEURO-IMMUNE-ENDOCRINE INTERFACE)

Exploring the intricate interplay between mind, body, and positive health necessitates a deep dive into the multifaceted realm of stress. Positive and negative stress are pivotal in shaping various physiological and psychological processes. Positive stress, termed eustress or hormesis, catalyses growth and adaptation, nurturing resilience against future challenges. Conversely, prolonged distress can detrimentally affect health, impacting immune function and cognitive abilities. By dissecting the mechanisms underlying stress responses, including the "fight or flight reaction" – the body's instinctive response to perceived threats – and the intricate roles of hormones and neurotransmitters, we unravel how our bodies navigate and react to stressors. Furthermore, understanding the delicate equilibrium between the sympathetic and parasympathetic nervous systems highlights the significance of relaxation and rejuvenation for overall wellbeing. In this context, delving into stress provides a panoramic view of the broader landscape of positive health and resilience.

One of the best ways to examine the complex interaction between the thinking process (psycho), the brain, the central nervous system (neuro), and the immune and hormone (endocrine) systems in the body is through the lens of stress (distress).

---

**Cold water** exposure is linked to increased dopamine, the neurotransmitter associated with pleasure, and the release of natural endorphins, which act as painkillers. The best part? You don't need to be a polar bear or dive into the sea to experience these benefits. Simply turning the shower dial to cold for 30 seconds at the end of a hot shower each morning can start benefiting you. Gradually increasing cold water exposure can yield surprising benefits and eventually feel good. The cold-water shock response, where we involuntarily gasp upon initial exposure, can be triggered by water as warm as 15°C, so you don't have to endure near-freezing temperatures to experience the hormetic effect.

---

Stress can be divided into brief or intermittent positive/beneficial stress (eustress and hormesis) (Mattson, 2008) and distress, which can be acute or chronic (sustained stress, experienced long-term) (Roberts & Karatsoreos, 2021). Without stress, it is unlikely that you would find the drive for self-improvement, education, or just getting up in the morning. Hormesis (from the Greek, *to excite*) is defined as a series of events whereby a living organism (single-celled, plant, or animal) is exposed to a low dose concentration of a chemical or environmental stressor that might cause harm at higher concentrations or exposure times, where the result is of benefit to the organism (Mattson, 2008). Hormesis has two phases, depending on the exposure and dose of the stressor. This leads to a U-shaped curve (inverted for potentially harmful stressors) when plotted on a graph (Calabrese, 2004). For example, controlled exposure to cold sea water for five minutes at a time (below 8°C) might benefit humans; however, falling overboard into a cold sea can cause hypothermia within ten minutes, which is highly harmful. Hormesis has received much attention recently, especially in association with cold water exposure and sea swimming (Harper, 2022). Exposing oneself to a controlled stressful situation can promote psychological and physical adaptation and growth, making the individual more resilient to future stressful events. The result can be enhanced resilience to similar future stressors (Li et al., 2019). Evidence emerging from research into the benefits of fasting and exercise describes positive impacts at a cellular level in metabolism and neurogenesis (developing new neurons in the brain), where the body adapts positively over time to controlled stressors (Calabrese & Mattson, 2017). However, it should be noted that Hormesis remains a largely theoretical construct and a hypothesis linked to developing resilience; much more research is required to confirm this concept as an essential part of health and wellbeing.

Stress can be associated with internal or external threats (perceived or physical) that trigger the fight or flight response. It is important to note that a similar fight or flight response can be triggered by (a) a real external threat, like a barking dog, or (b) an internal threat, such as worrying about losing your job. This is an essential point since we can often ignore the negative potential of persistent negative thinking and worry about the body.

The fight or flight response (Roberts & Karatsoreos, 2021) is associated with the release of chemicals (hormones and their precursors) into the bloodstream and the activation of the autonomic nervous system (ANS). The fight or flight response begins with an external or internal threat that activates the sympathetic nerves of the ANS. These nerves produce neurotransmitters such as adrenaline, released within seconds, causing increased blood pressure, heart rate, sweating, dilated pupils, tunnel vision, dry mouth, and limited higher-order thinking (associated with the brain's neocortex). Adrenaline also limits appetite and digestion, reduces libido and activates the anti-bacterial part of the immune system (Waxenbaum et al., 2023).

Hormones are chemical messengers involved with many functions, depending on where they are produced and their target organ. The hypothalamic–pituitary–adrenal (HPA) axis involves a cascade of hormones produced (starting in the brain) within minutes of any threat. Hormone precursors produced first in the hypothalamus (limbic brain) trigger the production of intermediate chemical messengers in the pituitary gland (also located in the limbic brain) that enter the bloodstream. Eventually, these messengers enter their target organ – the adrenal cortex (the inside part of the adrenal gland, which rests above both of your kidneys). The result is the production of the stress hormone cortisol. Cortisol has many functions; however, during a fight or flight response, its predominant role is to act in a negative feedback loop that limits the production of adrenaline and suppresses a potentially overactive immune response (Roberts & Karatsoreos, 2021).

Interestingly, the fight or flight response promotes a predominantly anti-bacterial immune response while simultaneously limiting the anti-viral immune arm (Irwin & Cole, 2011). This might be an evolutionary response to the prospect of our ancestors being bitten by an animal with a mouth teaming with life-threatening bacteria. Of course, you can see how chronic stress might render an individual susceptible to viral infection when it is sustained over a long period (Peters et al., 2021).

Notably, the sympathetic arm of the ANS has a corresponding inhibitory arm called the parasympathetic nervous system (PNS) associated with the *rest and digest* response. These nerves (predominantly the vagus nerve – cranial nerve X) emerge from the brain stem and the base of the spine. They are associated with the production of the neurotransmitter acetylcholine. Acetylcholine has many functions, including the capacity to act as an anti-inflammatory agent (Kelly et al., 2022; Matteoli & Boeckxstaens, 2013). The result is reduced breathing, heart rate, blood pressure, sweating, production of saliva, increased digestion and libido, emotional regulation and an improved capacity to focus with rational thinking (Bonaz et al., 2018).

## CHRONIC STRESS

Chronic stress can arise from distressing events, particularly when it persists over an undefined but prolonged period – a crucial factor being its sustained nature. While acute stress can serve a protective function against immediate threats, chronic stress can severely impact the body. This prolonged stress can present a spectrum of symptoms, highlighting the intricate connection between physical and mental health. If experiencing persistent symptoms, it is advisable to consult your GP or a local healthcare professional as the first step. Chronic stress symptoms encompass a wide range, including joint, tendon, and muscle discomfort, headaches, jaw tension and teeth grinding, sleep disturbances, fatigue, diminished pleasure, social withdrawal, appetite changes towards processed foods, concentration difficulties, emotional instability, irritability, decreased libido, gastrointestinal issues, itching, panic attacks, recurrent infections, reactivation of dormant viruses like the Varicella Zoster virus causing Shingles, and heightened alcohol consumption and/or drug use.

## STRESS MINDSETS

The significance of positive health in managing stress becomes apparent through the lens of stress mindsets, which highlight the profound influence of one's attitude toward stress on overall wellbeing. In a seminal study involving 28,753 US adults (Keller et al., 2012), researchers juxtaposed participants' stress levels with their beliefs regarding stress's impact on health, revealing a stark contrast in mortality rates eight years later: those who perceived stress as harmful faced a staggering 43% higher risk of premature death during periods of elevated stress, while those with heightened stress levels but a positive outlook experienced only an 8% increased risk. This study's pivotal finding highlights attitude's pivotal role in shaping stress's health effects. Over the past decade, abundant research has shed light on the tangible benefits of stress mindsets for overall wellbeing, extending beyond mere mortality statistics. Embracing a perspective that regards stress as potentially beneficial is a potent defence against its adverse effects. It empowers individuals to deploy more effective coping mechanisms and perceive stress as less menacing (Jenkins et al., 2021). This mindset has been demonstrated to alleviate symptoms of depression and anxiety within a month, fortify coping skills, and notably reduce somatic stress symptoms (Keech et al., 2021). Moreover, it correlated with improved cardiovascular health, the stimulation of growth-promoting hormones, enhanced physiological wellbeing, and resilience against heightened cortisol awakening responses (Silva et al., 2023). From a practical positive health standpoint, a stress-as-enhancer mindset is intricately linked to enhanced physiological, physical, and psychological wellbeing, rendering it a valuable concept to integrate into stress management approaches.

---

**Mindset** is one of humans' most powerful tools for improving their health. Researchers investigated whether individuals' beliefs about their physical activity could impact their physiological wellbeing. They recruited 84 female room attendants from various hotels and assessed their health metrics affected by exercise.

Participants in the informed group were informed that cleaning hotel rooms constituted valuable exercise, meeting the surgeon's recommendations for an active lifestyle. They provided concrete examples illustrating how their work contributed to the exercise. Conversely, individuals in the control group did not receive this information.

Remarkably, despite no observed change in their actual behaviour, those in the experimental group perceived themselves as engaging in significantly more exercise after four weeks. Consequently, compared to the control group, they exhibited weight, blood pressure, body fat, waist-to-hip ratio, and body mass index reductions. These findings demonstrated that our perception of our activity level can influence our health outcomes, highlighting the potency of mindset in shaping physical wellbeing (Crum & Langer, 2007).

---

During the COVID-19 pandemic, healthcare professionals who adopted a stress-is-enhancing mindset reported higher levels of posttraumatic growth compared to those with a stress-is-debilitating mindset (Zhang et al., 2023). This growth was supported by pro-active coping behaviours, such as reflecting on what caused them stress, asking for social support and directly addressing stressful situations. Similarly, research involving nurses showed a direct link between a stress-is-enhancing mindset, resilience, and, indirectly, mental health (Emirza & Yılmaz Kozcu, 2023). Introducing healthier stress mindsets can improve individuals' ability to manage their stressors effectively. These benefits can be realised through interventions designed to cultivate healthy mindsets and encourage a stress-as-enhancer perspective. In contrast, negative views of stress, often influenced by media portrayals, can lead to harmful coping behaviours such as symptom avoidance or substance use.

Two types of interventions have emerged to shift stress mindsets: stress reappraisal and stress mindset interventions. Stress reappraisal involves recognising stress responses as functional, viewing stress as a tool for active coping and a resource. This strategy aims to change individuals' perceptions of stress by encouraging them to see stress as a normal and even beneficial part of life. Stress mindset interventions, on the other hand, involve acknowledging both the positive and negative aspects of stress and embracing it to enhance performance. These interventions reduce attention to negative emotional stimuli, enhance cognitive flexibility, enable individuals to reassess their options, catalyse behavioural changes, and foster perceptions of greater resources. This leads to improved performance, elevated wellbeing, and persistence in pursuing personal goals. Understanding these intervention strategies can empower individuals to proactively reshape their stress mindsets.

Since the stress mindset is adaptable, diverse interventions have been deployed to modify it. For instance, many interventions have focused on educating participants about the positive impacts of stress through short videos or informational materials. These interventions aim to shift the perception of stress from a threat to a challenge, promoting a stress-as-enhancer mindset. A recent metacognitive approach has emerged, offering a balanced evaluation of stress by acknowledging both its positive and negative impacts (Crum et al., 2023). This holistic approach has improved physiological health outcomes beyond solely highlighting the benefits of stress. Therefore, a comprehensive consideration of both aspects of stress is essential for optimal results. Understanding and reshaping stress mindsets through tailored interventions is a crucial step that can make healthcare professionals feel more informed and prepared.

Understanding and reshaping stress mindsets through tailored interventions can pave the way for improved health outcomes and more effective coping strategies. This highlights the importance of adopting a positive perspective in managing stress effectively. Individuals can cultivate resilience, enhance wellbeing, and foster better teamwork in various professional settings by acknowledging stress as a potential enhancer rather than solely a detriment. Continued research and implementation of interventions aimed at promoting healthy stress mindsets can help individuals and communities thrive in the face of adversity, ultimately contributing to positive health outcomes on a broader scale.

## THE EPIGENOME: THE INTERFACE BETWEEN THE DNA IN EACH CELL OF YOUR BODY AND THE ENVIRONMENT

Thus far, we have described the (a) psycho–neuro–immune-endocrine and (b) microbiome interfaces that form part of the brain, mind, and body connection. Another critical interface is the epigenome, which internal and external environments can influence. Understanding the epigenome's role offers profound insights into positive health, highlighting how lifestyle, social, and physical environments can shape our genetic expressions without altering the DNA sequence. This dynamic interaction between genes and environment highlights the potential for positive health interventions to modify epigenetic marks, promoting wellbeing and resilience. By leveraging the knowledge of epigenetics, we can explore how behaviours, diets, and therapies can lead to beneficial epigenetic modifications, fostering improved health outcomes and enhanced quality of life.

Epigenetics studies how lifestyle, social, and physical environments can influence our genes; the prefix "epi" indicates something on, upon, above, or in addition to. An epigenetic trait is a heritable phenotype resulting from chromosome changes without changes in the DNA sequence (Shilatifard, 2009). The epigenome is a set of chemical instructions that help control our genes (NIEHS, 2024). These chemicals mark or tag our genes as on or off switches. Each cell in our body can have different marks on its DNA.

## INSIDE DNA

Before discussing epigenetic modifications, let's describe the structure of DNA inside cells. Accessing your genes is more complex than it seems. Under a microscope, the cell's most prominent structure is the nucleus, a "sphere within a sphere", which contains your DNA. One must first cross the nucleus barrier (membrane) to access the DNA. Inside the nucleus, DNA is tightly wrapped into structures resembling wool balls – this form is called chromatin (Figure 4.2). Chromatin is wrapped around large proteins called histones, with tails emerging at various points. These molecular tails are vital to unravelling the DNA. Adding acetyl molecules to these tails can unravel the DNA, making certain areas of the chromatin accessible while others remain closed. Different patterns or "marks" from attaching molecules like acetyl groups to histone tails are associated with biological functions and behaviours, such as anxiety (Bartlett et al., 2017).

When chromatin is unravelled using acetyl molecules, DNA is revealed in the form of chromosomes – humans have 23 pairs of chromosomes containing genes that provide the blueprint for human beings. A closer inspection of chromosomes shows DNA's exquisite double helix structure, composed of two strands bound in a helical structure. Even closer inspection reveals numerous coding sequences made of four repeating units called bases: adenosine (A), cytosine (C), guanine (G), and thymine (T). Different combinations of these four bases code for individual genes, each with a "start" and "stop" code. Some genes have a methyl ($CH_4$) molecule attached to the start code, silencing the gene. The amount of general methylation of DNA is associated with various biological functions and indirectly with lifestyle and behaviour (Hing et al., 2018). Acetylation of histones and methylation of DNA are the epigenetic modifications that have been studied the most.

## EPIGENETIC MODIFICATIONS

While direct evidence for transgenerational epigenetic inheritance in humans is lacking, some indirect evidence exists from long-term studies. Children and descendants of those who experienced the Dutch famine during the Second World War have shown an increased risk of obesity, glucose intolerance, and heart disease in adulthood.

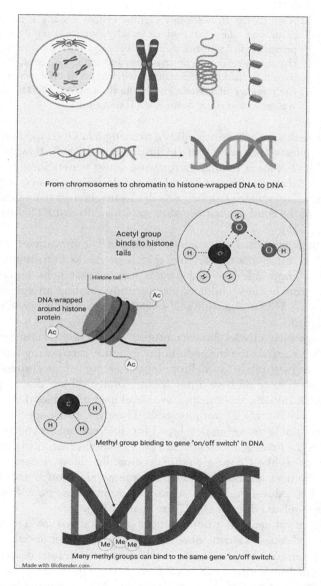

From chromosomes to chromatin to histone-wrapped DNA to DNA

Acetyl group binds to histone tails

Histone tail

DNA wrapped around histone protein

Methyl group binding to gene "on/off switch" in DNA

Many methyl groups can bind to the same gene "on/off switch."

Made with BioRender.com

*Figure 4.2* Epigenetic anatomy. The structure of chromosomes, DNA, and histones. DNA is found within the nucleus (top panel) of almost every cell in your body (the exception is the red blood cell).

(*Continued*)

*Figure 4.2* (Continued) In order to access the genetic code, it is necessary to unwrap chromatin, which is DNA wrapped tightly around proteins called histones. Addition of acetyl molecules can unravel chromatin to reveal chromosomes and individual genes (central panel). Individual genes can be switched on or off depending on the presence of a methyl molecule (bottom panel). This figure was generated using licensed BioRender software.

These health issues have been linked to changes in DNA methylation levels observed 70 years later (Heijmans et al., 2008). Researchers have also explored trauma transmission across generations, such as in the offspring of Second World War Holocaust survivors, combat veterans, and refugee families, revealing a heightened risk of mental illness in the third generation when grandparents had PTSD ((Raza et al., 2023).

Transgenerational epigenetic inheritance is controversial. Some scientists argue that transferring epigenetic marks from mother to child is impossible. Stressed parents may exhibit behaviours that cause stress in their children, subsequently creating an epigenetic mark for PTSD in the child's DNA rather than directly transferring these marks.

**Epigenetic clocks** allow scientists to create comprehensive maps of DNA methylation throughout the genome, monitoring biological ageing separately from chronological ageing (e.g., a chronological age of 50 could have a much older biological age due to poor lifestyle). Initially, these maps were developed using blood samples, describing the age of immune cells. However, tissue-specific epigenetic clocks are being developed for different organs and tissues, such as the brain (Grodstein et al., 2021). Advancements in epigenetic clocks, like GrimAge, estimate mortality, lifespan, and health span (Föhr et al., 2022). Epigenetic age acceleration is associated with low education, lower socio-economic status, poor lifestyle, and age-related diseases (McCrory et al., 2020).

The good news is that epigenetic modifications are reversible. Approved drugs can manipulate the epigenome of tumour cells, treating certain blood-borne cancers, such as with the histone deacetylase inhibitor drug Vorinostat (Yoon & Eom, 2016). This drug has also been examined in pre-clinical research, showing it can boost the immune response to Tuberculosis bacteria (Cox et al., 2020). Additionally, behaviour, lifestyle, and psychological therapies can influence epigenetic modification. One study showed cognitive behavioural therapy (CBT) could modify epigenetic patterns in genes related to the stress response (Roberts et al., 2015). Participants aged 5 to 18 across three study sites in Australia and the United Kingdom showed significant changes in the methylation status of the FKBP5 gene associated with the stress response after CBT exposure (Roberts et al., 2015).

Lorenzo and colleagues (Lorenzo et al., 2022) published a review describing the epigenetic impact of the Southern European Atlantic Diet, rich in fresh fruits and vegetables, olive oil, pulses, and nuts. Emerging evidence from animal studies suggests that exercise might positively impact the epigenome (Rasmussen et al., 2021). However, studies examining the impact of a healthy lifestyle on the epigenome have been mixed and need replication in humans. The jury is still out.

## VANTAGE SENSITIVITY

Vantage sensitivity theory posits that individuals vary in their responsiveness to positive experiences and interventions (Pluess et al., 2018). Some people who are vantage-sensitive benefit disproportionately from positive environmental influences, while others are vantage-resistant, and do not experience the same level of benefit from positive experiences. This theory extends the concept of differential susceptibility, which traditionally focused on individual responses to negative experiences, to include variability in reactions to positive experiences (Pluess & Belsky, 2013).

Vantage sensitivity, influenced by genetic, biological, and psychological factors, can be a game-changer. It makes some individuals more receptive to positive inputs, such as supportive relationships, beneficial therapies, positive health interventions, or enriching working or living environments. When exposed to positive influences, these sensitive individuals tend to show significant improvements in wellbeing, mental health, and overall functioning and their improvement lasts. This is a powerful testament to the potential of vantage sensitivity theory in improving health outcomes.

For example, a study involving young people undergoing psychological resilience training showed that 25% of individuals who were genetically predisposed to benefit from their environment experienced significant reductions in depression and anxiety symptoms immediately post-intervention and at six- and twelve-month follow-ups (Pluess & Boniwell, 2015). In contrast, vantage-resistant individuals, who were not genetically predisposed, showed improvement immediately post-intervention but no sustained improvement at six- or twelve-month follow-ups. These findings highlight why many positive health, positive psychology, or lifestyle medicine interventions often demonstrate only minor to medium impacts when outcomes are averaged across all participants. This averaging can obscure the reality that genetically predisposed vantage-resistant individuals may lower their overall scores while vantage-sensitive individuals continue to benefit disproportionately from interventions.

Understanding vantage sensitivity is crucial for tailoring tools and other interventions in positive health, positive psychology, and lifestyle medicine. This theory explains why some people experience substantial benefits from interventions while others show minimal improvement, highlighting the need for person-alised approaches to enhancing wellbeing and health outcomes. For instance, in positive health, this understanding could lead to developing more effective interventions for vulnerable individuals, thereby maximising their wellbeing. This could also explain why some individuals find it more difficult to maintain healthy weight than others, or why they pick up physical activity and develop a habit, whereas others struggle with it. Similarly, this knowledge could be used in positive health to design personalised lifestyle interventions that are more likely to yield positive health outcomes for each individual.

This finding also offers hope to everyone. Suppose you belong to a group of people genetically predisposed to be sensitive to their environment. In that case, the impact of positive health tools aimed at improving your nutrition, physical activity, or gratitude will be more profound and last longer. At the same time, if you belong to a group of individuals resistant to those interventions, you will still gain results. Still, they will not last as long, so you must engage in them more regularly to see sustained benefits. From an epigenetic point of view, we all can gain from these activities.

Understanding the epigenome's role offers profound insights into positive health, highlighting how lifestyle, social, and physical environments can shape our genetic expressions without altering the DNA sequence. Epigenetics explores how these environments influence our genes through chemical tags, acting as on/off switches for gene expression. DNA structure within cells reveals that accessing genetic information requires unwrapping chromatin, a process influenced by adding acetyl and methyl groups. These epigenetic modifications are linked to various biological functions and behaviours, such as anxiety. While the evidence for transgenerational epigenetic inheritance in humans remains controversial, studies suggest that environmental factors, such as famine or trauma, can impact DNA methylation and potentially influence future generations' health. Epigenetic clocks map DNA methylation and allow researchers to monitor biological ageing and its association with lifestyle factors. Importantly, epigenetic modifications are reversible, and interventions like drugs, diets, exercise, and psychological therapies have shown potential in promoting beneficial epigenetic changes. Leveraging this knowledge, positive health strategies can aim to enhance wellbeing and resilience through targeted lifestyle and therapeutic interventions.

### The O'Donnell family

*The O'Donnell family, part of the marginalised Irish Traveller community, face numerous challenges in terms of poor health, social stigma, and reduced access to education. The father, Steven, suffers from ill health, and struggles with chronic lung disease as a result of smoking cigarettes for over 20 years. His poor health is exacerbated by stress, a lack of access to quality healthcare and the fact that both he and his wife are unemployed. Sadly, both parents experienced PTSD in the form of violence in the family as young children. They are determined not to repeat this behaviour in their family.*

*The family met with a local social care worker (Emma) who uses vantage sensitivity theory as a means of supporting families to live healthier lives. She spoke with the O'Donnells about ways to leverage their environment and improve their wellbeing by being culturally* sensitive and respectful. The O'Donnells only have one smartphone and have low levels of literacy. Therefore, Emma had to find more accessible ways for the family to access support and education on health and wellbeing rather than through websites and apps.

Steven's wife, Mary, learned about the benefits of positive health interventions and decided to incorporate them into their daily lives. She started by improving the family diet, by introducing more fresh fruits and vegetables and reducing processed foods. It is a slow process but she finds that using humour and family competitions help with this gradual change. Their diet still isn't perfect but Steven eats far more vegetables (albeit only peas and carrots) than he used to. This has led to their children following suit. Steven is learning how to manage his conditions better.

Mary also encouraged daily physical activity. The family began taking walks together and engaging in physical activities that they enjoyed, like traditional Irish dance. These activities not only boosted their physical health but also provided emotional benefits, strengthening family bonds and improving her mood and fatigue.

Understanding the importance of supportive relationships, Mary fostered a sense of community within the wider Traveller community in the Leinster region. She organised regular gatherings where families could share meals and stories; the support and camaraderie really help. This social engagement proves vital in reducing stress and providing a network of emotional support. It's hard when you feel disconnected and marginalised.

Recognising the impact of their physical environment, the O'Donnells spend more time outdoors, connecting with nature. They found that exposure to natural surroundings has a calming effect and contributes to their physical and mental health. They spend time telling stories about dead loved ones (including pets and horses that were important to the family). The horse is very important in Irish Traveller culture, which helps the family engage positively with nature, as they look after these animals.

These positive changes, tailored to the family's unique sensitivities, led to significant improvements. Steven's health stabilised, his stress levels decreased, and the family experienced enhanced wellbeing. He has more confidence engaging with local healthcare support and is more willing to adhere to their advice. It is important that these local workers respect Steven, his family, and their traditions.

# ANTHROPOGENS, METAFLAMMATION, AND NCDS

## GERM THEORY

In today's world, we often take it for granted the idea that micro-organisms cause disease in humans and that basic hygiene could prevent the same illnesses. Yet, until the mid-1800s, this idea was considered radical and ground-breaking – a concept that became known as germ theory. Renowned scientists like Louis Pasteur, Joseph Lister, and Robert Koch are now synonymous with the development of antiseptic agents and antibiotics. They came to the conclusion that infectious diseases are often caused by microorganisms such as bacteria, viruses, fungi, and single-celled parasites like amoebae (Gaynes, 2011). We now know that eliminating or avoiding these disease-causing microorganisms (pathogens) will prevent infectious disease, a fact that has subsequently saved millions of lives through hygiene, antibiotics, and vaccines.

No equivalent of the germ theory has provided a satisfactory understanding of the origins of NCDs. Scientists argue that these chronic diseases can't be as a result of dysregulation caused by the aging process. The increase in the prevalence of chronic diseases and associated risk factors and behaviours among all age groups, limits aging as a sole explanation. Similarly, genetic influences and gene–age interactions are also incomplete explanations. Environmental factors have been implicated (early adverse childhood events, pollution and climate change), but a unifying, underlying theory has not been identified.

By recognising the transformative impact of germ theory on infectious diseases, we can strive for a similar breakthrough in understanding and addressing the root causes of NCDs. Just as hygiene practices and antibiotics have revolutionised public health, a deeper understanding of positive health factors and preventative measures may hold the key to combating the rise of chronic diseases and promoting overall wellbeing in society.

## ANTHROPOGENS AND METAFLAMMATION: A POTENTIAL UNIFYING THEORY FOR THE DEVELOPMENT OF NCDS

In 2012, Dr Garry Egger, an Australian academic and author, introduced a ground-breaking theory that has since captivated the field of public health. This theory, which links the surge in

NCDs with Western lifestyles and cultures, posits that the emergence of pro-inflammatory human-made products and processes since the Industrial Revolution has fuelled the rise in NCDs. Dr Egger's theory is not just a hypothesis but a compelling explanation backed by extensive research and evidence. He proposed that exposure to anthropogens, human-made or modified molecules capable of initiating immune responses, can induce a low-grade sub-clinical inflammation termed metaflammation (Egger et al., 2017) (Egger & Dixon, 2014).

Anthropogens, a diverse group of substances, can be found in various sources. Examples include by-products in tobacco smoke, air pollutants like sulphur dioxide, endocrine-disrupting chemicals in plastics, saturated fats, refined sugars in processed foods, pesticides, and fertilisers in polluted water (Egger & Dixon, 2014).

---

**LETTER OF GRATITUDE**

**(Moieni et al., 2019)**

Reflect on someone in your life whom you believe you've never adequately thanked for a meaningful deed. In the space below, compose a note to this individual explaining why you feel you need to express your gratitude adequately and detailing why you appreciate what they've done for you. While this letter won't be delivered to them and serves solely as an exercise, take this opportunity to delve deeply into your emotions regarding their actions and write sincerely and openly from your heart.

Research suggests that practicing gratitude once a week for six weeks led to decreases in inflammation.

---

Inflammation triggers the activation of immune cells, with human tissue releasing danger signals upon encountering anthropogens, such as excess low-density lipoprotein (LDL) in fast food. These signals prompt the release of cytokines, chemical messengers that recruit immune cells to sites of irritation or injury. This accumulation of immune cells can lead to plaque formation in arterial linings, culminating in atherosclerosis and potentially heart attacks if unchecked (Figure 4.3).

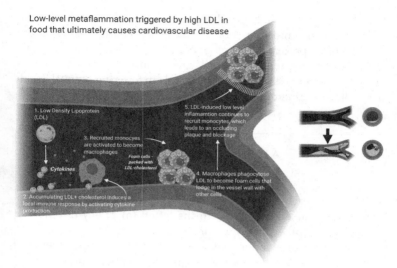

Low-level metaflammation triggered by high LDL in
food that ultimately causes cardiovascular disease

*Figure 4.3* Atherosclerosis caused by metaflammation. An example of an
anthropogens (LDL) found in processed food that if consumed
in enough quantities in conjunction with an inactive lifestyle,
can initiate metaflammation that ultimately leads to blockage of
an artery (atherosclerosis) and in some cases, heart attack. This
figure was generated using licensed BioRender software.

Unlike normal inflammation, which typically resolves within
days, metaflammation persists as the causative agents remain in the
system or individuals are continuously exposed to them through
diet or the environment. This type of anthropogen–induced inflammation, termed "metaflammation", is not just a health concern but
a chronic, low-grade, and systemic condition that can lead to various NCDs including obesity, chronic inflammation, dyslipidaemia,
insulin resistance, fatty liver disease, cardiovascular disease, respiratory issues, and certain cancers (Christ & Latz, 2019; Hotamisligil,
2017; Itoh et al., 2022; Kanbay et al., 2019). These are not just
words on a page but real health risks that we all need to be aware of
and take seriously.

While technological advances have led to the modification of
environmental molecules (anthropogens), triggering metaflammation, there is hope in recognising the role of positive health practices.

By promoting lifestyle habits that reduce exposure to anthropogens and mitigate inflammation, individuals can take control of their health and effectively prevent and manage NCDs. Embracing strategies such as a balanced diet, regular exercise, stress management, and environmental consciousness can play a pivotal role in fostering optimal health and wellbeing amidst the challenges posed by modern living.

---

### A LETTER OF FORGIVENESS

#### (Worthington Jr & Wade, 2020)

Take the next 30 minutes to compose a letter to someone who has caused you harm. In the letter, (a) briefly describe the event; (b) explain your understanding of the offender's motives; (c) outline the reasons for wanting to forgive them; and (d) explicitly state your forgiveness towards the individual who hurt or offended you.

Meta-analysis of research studies indicates that acts of forgiveness improve cardiovascular health, specifically heart-rate and blood pressure (Rasmussen et al., 2019).

---

## EMOTIONS AND INFLAMMATION

Negative emotions, moods, and traits have been associated with heightened levels of proinflammatory cytokines, which trigger inflammation in the body (Kiecolt-Glaser et al., 2002). For instance, individuals undergoing the Social Stress Task exhibited significantly elevated levels of proinflammatory cytokines and subsequent inflammation (Moons et al., 2010). Similarly, participants tasked with writing about self-blame on three occasions experienced increased proinflammatory cytokines (Dickerson et al., 2004). Therefore, situations that induce stress and lead to heightened negative emotions such as sadness, anger, frustration, loneliness, disappointment, fear, and guilt, among others, tend to elevate inflammation in the body.

Meanwhile, evidence suggests that positive emotions may have an inverse relationship with levels of proinflammatory cytokines. Generally, experiencing positive emotions is linked with increased longevity and reduced morbidity (Pressman & Cohen,

2005). Positive emotions are believed to expedite recovery from stress (Folkman & Moskowitz, 2000) and strengthen social connections (Fredrickson, 2004; Lyubomirsky et al., 2005), potentially leading to improved health and decreased inflammatory activity. The available literature provides evidence that positive affect correlates with reduced levels of proinflammatory cytokines. For example, optimism, often associated with heightened positive affect, predicts lower proinflammatory cytokine responses to stressors (Brydon et al., 2009), and watching a humorous film temporarily lowers proinflammatory cytokine levels (Mittwoch-Jaffe et al., 1995). Additionally, women reporting frequent extreme happiness throughout the day showed lower levels of proinflammatory cytokines (Steptoe et al., 2009). Furthermore, specific positive emotions like awe, measured in various ways, emerged as the strongest predictor of reduced proinflammatory cytokine levels.

In positive health, the convergence of lifestyle medicine, environmental factors, and the intricate interplay between the brain, mind, body, and microbiome offers a transformative approach to wellbeing. Recognising that our health is not solely determined by individual choices but also by the surrounding environment underscores the importance of holistic strategies. By nurturing harmony between ourselves and our surroundings, we unlock the full potential of positive health, transcending mere disease management to embrace physical vitality, mental resilience, and environmental balance. Through this lens, we embark on a journey toward thriving individuals and communities, empowered by the synergy between humanity and its environment.

### James' story

*James, a middle-aged man recently widowed, struggles with type 2 diabetes and experiences profound loneliness. The loss of his wife opened a deep emotional void, worsening his health. Formerly an optimistic person, he felt very negative toward life since the loss. Strangely, he has been contracting persistent viral infections; his doctor was also worried about increased inflammatory markers in blood, such as elevated c-reactive protein. Determined to make a change, James explored positive health practices through a friend who works in the local family resource centre.*

*James began by adopting a whole food, plant-based diet, focusing on foods that stabilised his blood sugar levels and his gut health.*

He was surprised at how much he took to the probiotic food, sauerkraut. His wife always made fun of his conservative approach to food – he never thought he would venture beyond the standard fare of spaghetti Bolognese, steak and potatoes, or the occasional fish and chips. James was not a friend of salads! He didn't get rid of his favourite foods but instead added small amounts of healthy greens, fibre (nuts and grains), fruit, and vegetables to meals each day. Some days he doesn't feel like eating healthily and that's OK.

He volunteered as a local scout leader since he has fond memories of being a scout as a young boy. This scared him as wasn't sure about how the children or other adults would react to him. He was also afraid of not being able to engage in the physical activities like hiking and camping. To address this fear, James committed to daily physical activity, starting with short walks that gradually became longer as his stamina improved. He loves showing the kids how to light fires and make camp tables using wood and fancy knots. The other leaders have commented on his natural way with the scouts, which has improved his confidence greatly.

Avoiding alcohol and processed foods further benefited his health. Living alone, he often drank too much alcohol and ate too much pizza in the evenings, often just to fill the emotional void in his life. He knew that was unhealthy but he couldn't seem to get out of the negative pattern.

The improved diet, and exercise, along with joining the scouts as a leader, eventually gave him the confidence to join a local support group for widowers. He somehow felt that this would be betraying his wife. However, these meetings filled another evening that might have been spent drinking alcohol alone. He liked to speak with other people who knew how he felt.

Although James is not ready to enter the dating world, he has adopted a dog, which not only provides companionship but also encourages him to stay active. He chats with locals in the park and in general feels better about himself. He would have never believed that these types of activities could improve his mood and general wellbeing, but they have.

Buoyed by these experiences, he decided to make a conscious effort to focus on what he had rather than what he had lost. He began with a gratitude journal that he added to on Sunday mornings.

Over time, James experienced significant improvements in his physical and mental health. His blood sugar levels stabilised, inflammatory

*markers reduced, his mood improved, and he felt more connected
and supported. By embracing positive health practices, James found
a pathway to healing and wellbeing, transforming his life after loss.*

## REFERENCES

ACLM. (2022). What is Lifestyle Medicine? www.lifestylemedicine.org/ ACLM/ACLM/About/What_is_Lifestyle_Medicine_/Lifestyle_Medicine. aspx?hkey=26f3eb6b-8294-4a63-83de-35d429c3bb88

Barrett, L. F. (2017). The theory of constructed emotion: An active inference account of interoception and categorization. *Social Cognitive and Affective Neuroscience, 12*(1), 1–23. https://doi.org/10.1093/scan/nsw154

Bartlett, A. A., Singh, R., & Hunter, R. G. (2017). Anxiety and epigenetics. *Advances in Experimental Medicine and Biology, 978*, 145–166. https://doi. org/10.1007/978-3-319-53889-1_8

Bonaz, B., Bazin, T., & Pellissier, S. (2018). The vagus nerve at the interface of the microbiota–gut–brain axis. *Frontiers in Neuroscience, 12*, 49. https://doi. org/10.3389/fnins.2018.00049

Bratman, G. N., Olvera-Alvarez, H. A., & Gross, J. J. (2021). The affective benefits of nature exposure. *Social and Personality Psychology Compass, 15*(8), e12630. https://doi.org/10.1111/spc3.12630

Brydon, L., Walker, C., Wawrzyniak, A., Whitehead, D., Okamura, H., Yajima, J., … Steptoe, A. (2009). Synergistic effects of psychological and immune stressors on inflammatory cytokine and sickness responses in humans. *Brain, Behavior, and Immunity, 23*(2), 217–224. https://doi.org/10.1016/j. bbi.2008.09.007

Burke, J., & Dunne, P. J. (2022). Lifestyle medicine pillars as predictors of psychological flourishing. *Frontiers in Psychology, 13*, 963806. https://doi. org/10.3389/fpsyg.2022.963806

Calabrese, E. J. (2004). Hormesis: a revolution in toxicology, risk assessment and medicine. *EMBO Rep, 5 Spec No*(Suppl 1), S37–S40. https://doi. org/10.1038/sj.embor.7400222

Calabrese, E. J., & Mattson, M. P. (2017). How does hormesis impact biology, toxicology, and medicine? *NPJ Aging and Mechanisms of Disease, 3*(1), 13. https://doi.org/10.1038/s41514-017-0013-z

Christ, A., & Latz, E. (2019). The Western lifestyle has lasting effects on metaflammation. *Nature Reviews Immunology, 19*(5), 267–268. https://doi. org/10.1038/s41577-019-0156-1

Cox, D. J., Coleman, A. M., Gogan, K. M., Phelan, J. J., Maoldomhnaigh, C. Ó., Dunne, P. J., … Keane, J. (2020). Inhibiting histone deacetylases in human macrophages promotes glycolysis, IL-1β and T helper cell responses to Mycobacterium tuberculosis. *Frontiers in Immunology, 11*, 1609.

Crum, A. J., & Langer, E. J. (2007). Mind-set matters: Exercise and the placebo effect. *Psychological Science*, *18*(2), 165–171. https://doi.org/10.1111/j.1467-9280.2007.01867.x

Crum, A. J., Santoro, E., Handley-Miner, I., Smith, E. N., Evans, K., Moraveji, N., ... Salovey, P. (2023). Evaluation of the "rethink stress" mindset intervention: A metacognitive approach to changing mindsets. *Journal of Experimental Psychology: General*, *152*(9), 2603–2622. https://doi.org/10.1037/xge0001396

Cryan, J. F., O'Riordan, K. J., Cowan, C. S. M., Sandhu, K. V., Bastiaanssen, T. F. S., Boehme, M., ... Dinan, T. G. (2019). The microbiota–gut–brain axis. *Physiological Reviews*, *99*(4), 1877–2013. https://doi.org/10.1152/physrev.00018.2018

Dickerson, S. S., Kemeny, M. E., Aziz, N., Kim, K. H., & Fahey, J. L. (2004). Immunological effects of induced shame and guilt. *Psychosomatic Medicine*, *66*(1), 124–131. https://doi.org/10.1097/01.psy.0000097338.75454.29

Egger, G., Binns, A., Rossner, S., & Sagner, M. (2017). *Lifestyle medicine* (3rd ed.). Academic Press.

Egger, G., & Dixon, J. (2014). Beyond obesity and lifestyle: A review of 21st century chronic disease determinants. *BioMed Research International*, *2014*, 731685–731685. https://doi.org/10.1155/2014/731685

Emirza, S., & Yılmaz Kozcu, G. (2023). Protecting healthcare workers' mental health against COVID-19-related stress: The effects of stress mindset and psychological resilience. *Nursing & Health Sciences*, *25*(2), 216–230. https://doi.org/10.1111/nhs.13018

Föhr, T., Törmäkangas, T., Lankila, H., Viljanen, A., Rantanen, T., Ollikainen, M., ... Sillanpää, E. (2022). The association between epigenetic clocks and physical functioning in older women: A 3-year follow-up. *Journals of Gerontology A: Biologival Sciences and Medical Sciences*, *77*(8), 1569–1576. https://doi.org/10.1093/gerona/glab270

Folkman, S., & Moskowitz, J. T. (2000). Positive affect and the other side of coping. *American Psychologist*, *55*(6), 647–654. https://doi.org/10.1037/0003-066X.55.6.647

Fredrickson, B. L. (2004). The broaden-and-build theory of positive emotions. *Philosophical Transactions of the Royal Society London B: Biologival Sciences*, *359*(1449), 1367–1378. https://doi.org/10.1098/rstb.2004.1512

Furman, D. J., Waugh, C. E., Bhattacharjee, K., Thompson, R. J., & Gotlib, I. H. (2013). Interoceptive awareness, positive affect, and decision making in major depressive disorder. *Journal of Affective Disorders*, *151*(2), 780–785. https://doi.org/10.1016/j.jad.2013.06.044

Gaynes, R. P. (2011). *Germ theory: Medical pioneers in infectious diseases*: ASM Press.

Grenham, S., Clarke, G., Cryan, J., & Dinan, T. (2011). Brain–gut–microbe communication in health and disease. *Frontiers in Physiology*, *2*(94). https://doi.org/10.3389/fphys.2011.00094

Grodstein, F., Lemos, B., Yu, L., Klein, H.-U., Iatrou, A., Buchman, A. S., ... Bennett, D. A. (2021). The association of epigenetic clocks in brain tissue with brain pathologies and common aging phenotypes. *Neurobiology of Disease*, *157*, 105428. https://doi.org/10.1016/j.nbd.2021.105428

Hansen, M. M., Jones, R., & Tocchini, K. (2017). Shinrin-yoku (forest bathing) and nature therapy: A state-of-the-art review. *International Journal of Environmental Research and Public Health*, *14*(8). https://doi.org/10.3390/ijerph14080851

Harper, M. (2022). *Chill: The cold water swim cure – a transformative guide to renew your body and mind*. Chronicle Books.

Hefferon, K. (2013). *Positive psychology and the body: The somatopsychic side to flourishing*. Open University Press.

Heijmans, B. T., Tobi, E. W., Stein, A. D., Putter, H., Blauw, G. J., Susser, E. S., ... Lumey, L. H. (2008). Persistent epigenetic differences associated with prenatal exposure to famine in humans. *Proceedings of the National Academy of Sciences of the United States of America*, *105*(44), 17046–17049. https://doi.org/10.1073/pnas.0806560105

Hing, B., Braun, P., Cordner, Z. A., Ewald, E. R., Moody, L., McKane, M., ... Potash, J. B. (2018). Chronic social stress induces DNA methylation changes at an evolutionary conserved intergenic region in chromosome X. *Epigenetics*, *13*(6), 627–641. https://doi.org/10.1080/15592294.2018.1486654

Hotamisligil, G. S. (2017). Inflammation, metaflammation and immunometabolic disorders. *Nature*, *542*(7640), 177–185. https://doi.org/10.1038/nature21363

Irwin, M. R., & Cole, S. W. (2011). Reciprocal regulation of the neural and innate immune systems. *Nature Reviews Immunology*, *11*(9), 625–632. https://doi.org/10.1038/nri3042

Itoh, H., Ueda, M., Suzuki, M., & Kohmura-Kobayashi, Y. (2022). Developmental origins of metaflammation: A bridge to the future between the DOHaD theory and evolutionary biology. *Front Endocrinol (Lausanne)*, *13*, 839436. https://doi.org/10.3389/fendo.2022.839436

Jain, N. (2020). The early life education of the immune system: Moms, microbes and (missed) opportunities. *Gut Microbes*, *12*(1), 1824564. https://doi.org/10.1080/19490976.2020.1824564

Jenkins, A., Weeks, M. S., & Hard, B. M. (2021). General and specific stress mindsets: Links with college student health and academic performance. *PLOS ONE*, *16*(9), e0256351. https://doi.org/10.1371/journal.pone.0256351

Kanbay, M., Yerlikaya, A., Sag, A. A., Ortiz, A., Kuwabara, M., Covic, A., … Afsar, B. (2019). A journey from microenvironment to macroenvironment: the role of metaflammation and epigenetic changes in cardiorenal disease. *Clinical Kidney Journal*, *12*(6), 861–870. https://doi.org/10.1093/ckj/sfz106

Keech, J. J., Orbell, S., Hagger, M. S., O'Callaghan, F. V., & Hamilton, K. (2021). Psychometric properties of the stress control mindset measure in university students from Australia and the UK. *Brain Behavior*, *11*(2), e01963. https://doi.org/10.1002/brb3.1963

Keller, A., Litzelman, K., Wisk, L. E., Maddox, T., Cheng, E. R., Creswell, P. D., & Witt, W. P. (2012). Does the perception that stress affects health matter? The association with health and mortality. *Health Psychology*, *31*(5), 677–684. https://doi.org/10.1037/a0026743

Kelly, M. J., Breathnach, C., Tracey, K. J., & Donnelly, S. C. (2022). Manipulation of the inflammatory reflex as a therapeutic strategy. *Cell Reports Medicine*, *3*(7), 100696. https://doi.org/10.1016/j.xcrm.2022.100696

Khalsa, S. S., Adolphs, R., Cameron, O. G., Critchley, H. D., Davenport, P. W., Feinstein, J. S., … Paulus, M. P. (2018). Interoception and mental health: A roadmap. *Biological Psychiatry: Cognitive Neuroscience and Neuroimaging*, *3*(6), 501–513. https://doi.org/10.1016/j.bpsc.2017.12.004

Kiecolt-Glaser, J. K., McGuire, L., Robles, T. F., & Glaser, R. (2002). Psychoneuroimmunology: Psychological influences on immune function and health. *Journal of Consulting and Clinical Psychology*, *70*(3), 537–547. https://doi.org/10.1037//0022-006x.70.3.537

Li, X., Yang, T., & Sun, Z. (2019). Hormesis in health and chronic diseases. *Trends in Endocrinology & Metabolism*, *30*(12), 944–958. https://doi.org/10.1016/j.tem.2019.08.007

Lianov, L., & Burke, J. (2023). Positive psychology approaches to mental health and health behaviour interventions. In G. Merlo & C. P. P. Fagundes (Eds.), *Lifestyle psychiatry: Through the lens of behavioural medicine (Lifestyle Medicine)*. CRC Press.

Lorenzo, P. M., Izquierdo, A. G., Rodriguez-Carnero, G., Fernández-Pombo, A., Iglesias, A., Carreira, M. C., … Crujeiras, A. B. (2022). Epigenetic effects of healthy foods and lifestyle habits from the southern European Atlantic diet pattern: A narrative review. *Advances in Nutrition*, *13*(5), 1725–1747. https://doi.org/10.1093/advances/nmac038

Lyubomirsky, S., King, L., & Diener, E. (2005). The benefits of frequent positive affect: Does happiness lead to success? *Psychological Bulletin*, *131*(6), 803–855. https://doi.org/10.1037/0033-2909.131.6.803

Matteoli, G., & Boeckxstaens, G. E. (2013). The vagal innervation of the gut and immune homeostasis. *Gut*, *62*(8), 1214–1222. https://doi.org/10.1136/gutjnl-2012-302550

Mattson, M. P. (2008). Dietary factors, hormesis and health. *Ageing Research Review*, *7*(1), 43–48. https://doi.org/10.1016/j.arr.2007.08.004

McCrory, C., Fiorito, G., Hernandez, B., Polidoro, S., O'Halloran, A. M., Hever, A., … Kenny, R. A. (2020). GrimAge outperforms other epigenetic clocks in the prediction of age-related clinical phenotypes and all-cause mortality. *The Journals of Gerontology: Series A*, *76*(5), 741–749. https://doi.org/10.1093/gerona/glaa286 %J

McGilchrist, I. (2012). *The master and his emissary: The divided brain and the making of the western world*. Yale University Press.

Mittwoch-Jaffe, T., Shalit, F., Srendi, B., & Yehuda, S. (1995). Modification of cytokine secretion following mild emotional stimuli. *Neuroreport*, *6*(5), 789–792. https://doi.org/10.1097/00001756-199503270-00021

Moieni, M., Irwin, M. R., Haltom, K. E. B., Jevtic, I., Meyer, M. L., Breen, E. C., … Eisenberger, N. I. (2019). Exploring the role of gratitude and support-giving on inflammatory outcomes. *Emotion*, *19*(6), 939–949. https://doi.org/10.1037/emo0000472

Moons, W. G., Eisenberger, N. I., & Taylor, S. E. (2010). Anger and fear responses to stress have different biological profiles. *Brain, Behavior, and Immunity*, *24*(2), 215–219. https://doi.org/10.1016/j.bbi.2009.08.009

NIEHS (2024). Epigenetics. www.niehs.nih.gov/health/topics/science/epigenetics

Peters, E. M. J., Schedlowski, M., Watzl, C., & Gimsa, U. (2021). To stress or not to stress: Brain–behavior–immune interaction may weaken or promote the immune response to SARS-CoV-2. *Neurobiology of Stress*, *14*, 100296. https://doi.org/10.1016/j.ynstr.2021.100296

Pfefferle, P. I., Keber, C. U., Cohen, R. M., & Garn, H. (2021). The hygiene hypothesis: Learning from but not living in the past. *Frontiers in Immunology*, *12*, 635935. https://doi.org/10.3389/fimmu.2021.635935

Piran, N. (2016). Embodied possibilities and disruptions: The emergence of the Experience of Embodiment construct from qualitative studies with girls and women. *Body Image*, *18*, 43–60. https://doi.org/10.1016/j.bodyim.2016.04.007

Piran, N., Teall, T. L., & Counsell, A. (2020). The experience of embodiment scale: Development and psychometric evaluation. *Body Image*, *34*, 117–134. https://doi.org/10.1016/j.bodyim.2020.05.007

Pluess, M., Assary, E., Lionetti, F., Lester, K. J., Krapohl, E., Aron, E. N., & Aron, A. (2018). Environmental sensitivity in children: Development of the Highly Sensitive Child Scale and identification of sensitivity groups. *Developmental Psychology*, *54*(1), 51–70. https://doi.org/10.1037/dev0000406

Pluess, M., & Belsky, J. (2013). Vantage sensitivity: Individual differences in response to positive experiences. *Psychological Bulletin*, *139*(4), 901–916. https://doi.org/10.1037/a0030196

Pluess, M., & Boniwell, I. (2015). Sensory-Processing Sensitivity predicts treatment response to a school-based depression prevention program: Evidence of Vantage Sensitivity. *Personality and Individual Differences*, *82*, 40–45. https://doi.org/10.1016/j.paid.2015.03.011

Pressman, S. D., & Cohen, S. (2005). Does positive affect influence health? *Psychological Bulletin, 131*(6), 925–971. https://doi.org/10.1037/0033-2909.131.6.925

Rasmussen, K. R., Stackhouse, M., Boon, S. D., Comstock, K., & Ross, R. (2019). Meta-analytic connections between forgiveness and health: The moderating effects of forgiveness-related distinctions. *Psychological Health, 34*(5), 515–534. https://doi.org/10.1080/08870446.2018.1545906

Rasmussen, L., Knorr, S., Antoniussen, C. S., Bruun, J. M., Ovesen, P. G., Fuglsang, J., & Kampmann, U. (2021). The impact of lifestyle, diet and physical activity on epigenetic changes in the offspring-a systematic review. *Nutrients, 13*(8). https://doi.org/10.3390/nu13082821

Raza, Z., Hussain, S. F., Foster, V. S., Wall, J., Coffey, P. J., Martin, J. F., & Gomes, R. S. M. (2023). Exposure to war and conflict: The individual and inherited epigenetic effects on health, with a focus on post-traumatic stress disorder. *Frontiers in Epidemiology, 3.* https://doi.org/10.3389/fepid.2023.1066158

Roberts, B. L., & Karatsoreos, I. N. (2021). Brain–body responses to chronic stress: A brief review. *Faculty Reviews, 10*, 83. https://doi.org/10.12703/r/10-83

Roberts, S., Keers, R., Lester, K. J., Coleman, J. R., Breen, G., Arendt, K., ... Wong, C. C. (2015). HPA axis related genes and response to psychological therapies: Genetics and epigenetics. *Depress Anxiety, 32*(12), 861–870. https://doi.org/10.1002/da.22430

Shilatifard, A. (2009). Definition of 'epigenetics' clarified. www.sciencedaily.com/releases/2009/04/090401181447.htm

Silva, F. C., Ferreira de Jesus, M. C., & Souza-Talarico, J. N. (2023). Stress-is-debilitating mindset is linked to higher cortisol awakening response in women. *Psychoneuroendocrinology, 153*, 106228. https://doi.org/10.1016/j.psyneuen.2023.106228

Slotta, T., Witthöft, M., Gerlach, A. L., & Pohl, A. (2021). The interplay of interoceptive accuracy, facets of interoceptive sensibility, and trait anxiety: A network analysis. *Personality and Individual Differences, 183*, 111133. https://doi.org/10.1016/j.paid.2021.111133

Steptoe, A., Dockray, S., & Wardle, J. (2009). Positive affect and psychobiological processes relevant to health. *Journal of Personality, 77*(6), 1747–1776. https://doi.org/10.1111/j.1467-6494.2009.00599.x

Thibaut, F. (2018). The mind–body Cartesian dualism and psychiatry. *Dialogues in Clinical Neuroscience, 20*(1), 3. https://doi.org/10.31887/DCNS.2018.20.1/fthibaut

Tylka, T. L., & Kroon Van Diest, A. M. (2013). The Intuitive Eating Scale-2: Item refinement and psychometric evaluation with college women and men. *Journal of Counseling Psychology, 60*(1), 137–153. https://doi.org/10.1037/a0030893

Ursell, L. K., Metcalf, J. L., Parfrey, L. W., & Knight, R. (2012). Defining the human microbiome. *Nutrition Reviews, 70 Suppl 1*(Suppl 1), S38–S44. https://doi.org/10.1111/j.1753-4887.2012.00493.x

Waxenbaum, J. A., Reddy, V., & Varacallo, M. (2023). *Anatomy, autonomic nervous system.* www.ncbi.nlm.nih.gov/books/NBK539845/

WHO. (2021, 21-04-21). Noncommunicable diseases (Key Facts). www.who.int/news-room/fact-sheets/detail/noncommunicable-diseases#:~:text=Noncommunicable%20diseases%20(NCDs)%20kill%2041,%2D%20and%20middle%2Dincome%20countries

Worthington Jr, E. L., & Wade, N. G. (2020). A new perspective on forgiveness research. In *Handbook of forgiveness* (2nd ed.; pp. 345–355). Routledge.

Yoon, S., & Eom, G. H. (2016). HDAC and HDAC Inhibitor: From cancer to cardiovascular diseases. *Chonnam Medical Journal, 52*(1), 1–11. https://doi.org/10.4068/cmj.2016.52.1.1

Zhang, N., Bai, B., & Zhu, J. (2023). Stress mindset, proactive coping behavior, and posttraumatic growth among health care professionals during the COVID-19 pandemic. *Psychological Trauma: Theory, Research, Practice, and Policy, 15*(3), 515–523. https://doi.org/10.1037/tra0001377

# POSITIVE HEALTH WITHIN THE PILLARS OF LIFESTYLE MEDICINE

Lifestyle medicine represents an integral arm of positive health sciences. Therefore, it is important to provide a summary of its inception, and current place in healthcare and medicine. An old concept, largely forged from common sense practices, its modern iteration has been developed as a tool to promote a healthy lifestyle and prevent the treatment of chronic disease (ACLM, 2022). It is also important to provide a detailed account of the best-practice recommendations on how to live a healthy life, which are provided by some of the world's most trusted organisations such as the WHO (WHO, 2020). For this reason, you will find a detailed description of these guidelines under each pillar. This essential research-based information can then act as a foundation upon which to add positive health interventions that can be sampled independently or delivered via positive health coaches. Studies investigating the health-promoting capacity of positive psychology interventions and lifestyle medicine practices, as a combined positive health approach are still relatively small in number. However, the emerging findings point to the fact that combined interventions might act synergistically to improve health and wellbeing, promote flourishing, and even prevent the development of disease (Burke & Dunne, 2022; Lianov & Burke, 2025).

## LESSONS FROM GEOGRAPHICAL LOCATIONS WHERE HUMANS LIVE THE LONGEST IN GOOD HEALTH

Back in the early 2000s, Dan Buettner, in collaboration with scientists and demographers from National Geographic, set out on

DOI: 10.4324/9781003457169-5

a journey to explore what they would later term the blue zones (Buettner, 2012). Blue zones are regions where people live significantly longer than the global average. The story behind the name is equally intriguing: these areas were marked on a world map with a blue marker, hence the name. The first five blue zones identified were Loma Linda (California, US), Nicoya Peninsula (Costa Rica), Nuoro Province (Sardinia, Italy), Ikaria (Greece), and Okinawa (Japan).

A striking contrast emerges when examining longevity data from various nations alongside those from the blue zones (Table 5.1). In 2022, just over nine individuals (9.3) per 100,000 Irish citizens reached 100 or older, according to the Central Statistics Office of Ireland (CSO, 2022). In contrast, the Nuoro Province of Sardinia boasted 17.9 centenarians per 100,000 inhabitants in 2013 (Poulain et al., 2013). Even more striking is the gender distribution among centenarians: in Ireland, there is a ratio of five women to every man who reaches 100 years or beyond, as reported by the Central Statistics Office (CSO) of Ireland, while in the Nuoro Province, it is a 1:1 ratio (Table 5.1) (Poulain et al., 2013). This parity in life expectancy between men and women is a rarity across global regions, further highlighting the unique characteristics of the blue zones.

*Table 5.1* Number of people who live to be 100 years and older, as well as the ratio of women to men living to this age in European countries and the Nuoro Province (blue zone), Sardinia

| Country/Region | Number of people who live to 100 years per 100,000 population | Ratio of women to men who live to be 100 years and older |
| --- | --- | --- |
| **Ireland** | 9.3* | 5:1* |
| **Sweden** | 12.6 | 6:1 |
| **Italy** | 14.1 | 4:1 |
| **Sardinia** | 16.6 | 3:1 |
| **Nuoro Province, Sardinia** | 17.9 | 1:1 |

Source: *CSO Ireland. The other statistics are sourced from Michael Poulain, Ann Herm, and Gianni Pes, *Vienna Yearbook of Population Research 2013* (Vol. 11), pp. 87–108.

## WHAT DO THE BLUE ZONES HAVE IN COMMON?

### BEHAVIOURAL AND GENETIC ASSOCIATIONS

The standard practices observed in blue zone communities that foster longevity include natural movement beyond structured exercise routines, resilience to stress, strong family and community bonds, and a deep sense of purpose and meaning in life (Kreouzi et al., 2022).

In their analysis, Kreouzi and colleagues noted the significance of genetic factors in understanding longevity (Kreouzi et al., 2022). They highlighted several interesting genes, including FOXO3A, recognised as a tumour suppressor gene; Apolipoprotein E2, potentially linked to neuronal health and protecting against Alzheimer's disease; and Human Leucocyte Antigen genes, which have associations with some types of autoimmune disease (Kreouzi et al., 2022). However, despite these insights, the quest for a definitive "longevity gene" shared by inhabitants of blue zones remains elusive. Perhaps we should delve deeper into epigenetics, to explore whether these individuals share distinct epigenetic profiles that set them apart from the broader population.

**Life span and health span**: It is essential to be able to differentiate these two phrases. This is especially the case in the 21st century when we live longer but do not necessarily have a higher quality of life. In fact, according to a 2022 report by the McKinsey Health Institute ("Adding years to life and life to years"), although life spans have increased globally since the 1960s (54 versus 73 years), health spans have primarily stayed the same at 54 years (McKinsey, 2022). According to the *Oxford Languages Dictionary*: (1) **Life span** is the length of time for which a person or animal lives or a thing functions, while (2) **Health span** represents the part of a person's life during which they are generally in good health. One of the goals of positive health Science is to find evidence-based, multidisciplinary approaches to promoting longer health spans among our communities. We must strive to develop strategies on a global level that support all humans to live long into old age without significant suffering and ill health.

## LIFESTYLE CHARACTERISTICS

Poulain and colleagues (Poulain et al., 2013) have identified the significance of daily physical activity engagement, the adoption of stress-reducing habits, and strong community support among enduring inhabitants of blue zones, particularly in regions like the Nuoro Province and Okinawa. These elements are considered pivotal factors contributing to longevity and extended periods of good health.

## DIETARY HABITS

The dietary practices of blue zone inhabitants primarily revolve around whole, plant-based foods, a pattern associated with lower rates of chronic disease and supporting longevity (Pes et al., 2022). Typical blue zone diets include whole grain cereals, legumes, nuts, locally sourced olive oil, and abundant fresh fruits and vegetables. This fresh produce is predominantly sourced locally, often making a direct journey from garden to table or, at most, from market to table. Although blue zone communities eat a mostly plant-based diet, meat is not excluded entirely. Most people consume meat, fish, and dairy products, particularly goats, over cows, every week.

## PSYCHOLOGICAL CHARACTERISTICS

Studies highlight the positive psychological traits observed among elderly individuals residing in the Sardinian blue zone, particularly in the Nuoro Province, including lower rates of depression and heightened self-reported wellbeing, which seem to contribute to their extended lifespan (Hitchcott et al., 2018). Moreover, individuals in these regions, especially Loma Linda, Costa Rica, Ikaria, and Greece, share a strong religious faith compared to their geographical neighbours. These aspects may contribute to greater psychological health and a profound sense of wellbeing among these populations (Hitchcott et al., 2018).

In summary, the current findings suggest that the factors associated with longevity in the five most extensively studied blue zones emphasise a combination of lifestyle choices, community support, diet, and psychological wellbeing. Remarkably, these elements align closely with the pillars of lifestyle medicine.

## CRITICISM OF BLUE ZONE STUDIES AND THE BLUE ZONE MOVEMENT

The blue zones model, a significant paradigm in the fields of gerontology (study of ageing) and public health, has not been without its share of academic critiques. In 2024, Saul Justin Newman (Newman, 2024), a renowned gerontologist, published a critique of the blue zone initiative and studies. According to Newman, less than 20% of fully evaluated supercentenarians (those who live longer than 100 years) living in blue zone countries have a birth certificate; this number drops to zero per cent in America. Newman also noted that supercentenarian birth dates are recorded on days divisible by five, a numerical pattern indicative of either fraud or error. Rather than being associated with long life and health spans, Newman suggests that being a supercentenarian (especially in Okinawa and Sardinia) is actually associated with low income and literacy rates, high crime rates and short life expectancy, relative to the national averages recorded in Japan and Italy, respectively.

Buettner, in his response to these criticisms (Buettner, 2024), highlights the meticulousness of the original researchers, demographers, and scientists who personally visited each blue zone region to validate the age of supercentenarians. This involved cross-referencing birth certificates with church baptism records or other available local records. Buettner also counters Newman's claim that the blue zones are areas with the most supercentenarians, stating that they are regions with the highest health spans, where people reach their nineties with low rates of chronic disease; the probability of reaching 100 is significantly higher in these regions. Lastly, Buettner acknowledged that certain blue zones, like those in Sardinia, are among the poorer regions of Italy. However, he asserted that they are also places where modernisation and the Western diet have been slower to take hold (Buettner, 2024).

**Cultural and genetic factors**. Some critics argue that Buettner's conclusions often oversimplify the complex interplay of genetic, environmental, and cultural factors contributing to longevity. For example, a population's genetic makeup can significantly influence health outcomes (inbreeding can occur in some isolated geographical regions). It may not apply to people outside that genetic pool.

**Economic and social determinants of health**. The blue zones model sometimes underestimates the role of socio-economic status and healthcare access in determining longevity. These factors can vary widely between and within countries, influencing health outcomes independently of the lifestyle choices emphasised by Dan Buettner and blue zone-related scientists.

**Media and commercial interests**. Dan Buettner's work has been extensively commercialised, leading to potential conflicts of interest. The branding of the blue zones has led to partnerships with various health and wellness products, which might detract from the scientific rigour and objectivity of the findings.

**Simplistic health messages**. The popularisation of the blue zones has occasionally led to the delivery of simplistic health messages. For example, promoting specific blue zone diets or lifestyle choices as a panacea for longevity overlooks the more complex health narratives needed for diverse populations with different health profiles. Remember, there is rarely a one-size-fits-all approach for humans, especially regarding health and wellbeing.

While the concept of the blue zones offers valuable insights into factors that contribute to longevity, a more nuanced approach is required in future research. Acknowledging the complex interdependencies of lifestyle, genetics, environment, political landscape, and social structures will enhance the accuracy of longevity studies inspired by the blue zones. Regardless of the complexity and critiques, the blue zone initiative has pointed us toward a positive health science approach that applies positive psychology-based interventions and lifestyle medicine-based practices for better health. The need for trustworthy, evidence-based research and dissemination for preventing, treating, and managing noncommunicable diseases has never been more relevant.

## THE PILLARS OF LIFESTYLE MEDICINE

### SLEEP

The American National Sleep Foundation published an updated report in 2015 on recommended sleep durations for healthy individuals of all ages (Hirshkowitz et al., 2015). Their recommendations are as follows: 14–17 hours for new-borns, 12–15 hours for infants, 11–14 hours for toddlers, 10–13 hours for pre-schoolers,

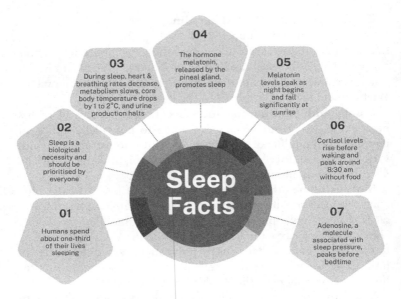

*Figure 5.1* Seven facts about sleep.

9–11 hours for school children, and 8–10 hours for teenagers. For young adults and adults, 7–9 hours per night is recommended, while older adults should aim for 7–8 hours (Hirshkowitz et al., 2015). Prioritising sleep within the framework of positive health is essential for overall wellbeing and vitality. For more facts about sleep, go to Figure 5.1.

## CIRCADIAN RHYTHM

Living beings on Earth experience a natural rhythm of day and night that is controlled by internal biological clocks, which can be influenced by external factors, including lifestyle practices (Patke et al., 2020). The human circadian rhythm is 24.2 hours long, meaning that whether you were exposed to daylight or spent life in a cave, your internal physiology would behave as if night came during each cycle (Czeisler & Gooley, 2007). Research indicates that this rhythm is controlled by an internal biological clock, primarily situated in two regions of the brain known as the suprachiasmatic nuclei, particularly in mammals. These nuclei, often the focus of our research, play a crucial role in regulating our sleep-wake cycle (Patke et al., 2020). During normal day/ night cycles, daylight reaching the back of the eye, stimulates the optic nerve, which in turn activates the suprachiasmatic nucleus (SCN). The SCN is the master clock in the brain that governs the production of the hormone melatonin by the pineal gland. Melatonin is entrained in the light/dark cycle (i.e. trained by daylight and darkness at night time) and helps to synchronise internal body systems in relation to the outside world, especially light.

When it comes to the connection between circadian rhythms and overall wellbeing, individuals who are morning people (larks) often report higher levels of happiness compared to evening people (owls). Various studies, such as those by Gobinath (Gobinath & Jothimani, 2020) and Tan (Tan et al., 2020), have used a range of happiness and wellbeing measures to assess this phenomenon. Some researchers even suggest that the higher incidence of positive emotions experienced by individuals over 55 years, in contrast to younger individuals, may be linked to their tendency towards waking early (Biss & Hasher, 2012).

At the Centre for positive health Sciences, we are currently investigating the effects of positive health interventions implemented at different times throughout the day. We aim to determine whether specific times offer particular benefits for both larks and owls in enhancing their wellbeing. Thus, circadian rhythm should not be disregarded in the context of positive health.

## SLEEP CYCLES

Each sleep cycle is a natural and necessary process that occurs in five stages. These stages include the waking state, three stages of non-rapid eye movement (REM) sleep that start with light and progress to deep sleep, and finally, rapid eye movement (REM) sleep, where we often dream (Patel et al., 2024). It's reassuring to know that most individuals experience 4 to 6 sleep cycles each night, typically lasting between 90 to 110 minutes. During the first cycle, REM is short; however, as the night progresses, longer periods of REM occur. This is why we often recall our dreams just after waking in the morning. Deep sleep (NREM) is crucial for recovery and growth, a functioning immune system (Yordanova et al., 2010), creativity (Drago et al., 2011), and memory (Antony et al., 2019). Dream sleep (REM) is associated with atonia (paralysis except for breathing and eye movement), learning, faster cognition (Peever & Fuller, 2016), and reducing fear and anxiety by consolidating memories (Ai & Dai, 2018).

### ZEITGEBERS (TIME GIVERS)

The internal circadian rhythm moves independently of external factors (e.g. if you stayed in a cave for 30 days, your circadian rhythm would be intact). However, it can be synchronised with external factors called Zeitgebers (time givers) (Schulz et al., 1997). Common zeitgebers include light, ambient temperature, food and feeding times, blood flow and water intake, and physical activity. Sleep and circadian rhythm can be entrained by modifying these zeitgebers (Schulz & Steimer, 2009). External zeitgebers can influence sleep or be influenced by sleep deficits in many ways (Table 5.2); modifying these external factors is essential to getting adequate, healthy sleep. Any disturbances to these biological rhythms can harm the organism's overall health and wellbeing.

### SLEEP AND WELLBEING

We intuitively understand that sleep benefits our wellbeing, but it is important to explore the scientific research between sleep and positive health outcomes. From an emotional viewpoint, the process of falling asleep, the duration, and the quality of sleep are closely

*Table 5.2* Zeitgebers (time givers) represent external factors that can be used to entrain (train or modify) sleep

| Zeitgeber | Facts |
| --- | --- |
| **Light** | • Daylight exposure suppresses melatonin and promotes alertness<br>• Shortwave blue light (420–480 nm) creates greater melatonin suppression even at short durations. E.g. smartphone, tablet, computer and TV screens<br>• Longwave warm red light (700 nm) is more conducive to sleep, e.g. fire flame<br>• Blue light increases heart rate, blood pressure, core body temperature, sympathetic tone, and alertness |
| **Food** | • Good sleep lowers cortisol and blood glucose, increases insulin sensitivity and leptin (appetite suppression), and reduces food-seeking behaviour<br>• Consuming carbohydrates late at night delays sleep onset<br>• Eating a carbohydrate-rich dinner too early leads to early (unwanted) sleep onset |
| **Exercise** | • Morning and afternoon exercise help with the transition from wakefulness to sleep at night<br>• Evening exercise delays sleep onset<br>• Exercise promotes thermoregulation (warming and cooling of the core temperature)<br>• Exercise in the day leads to a gradual increase in adenosine, which contributes to sleep pressure |
| **Fluid intake** | • Increased skin temperature at night is associated with a parallel low core temperature – fluid in the blood stream affects skin temperature<br>• High sodium (salt) meals will lead to an eventual increase in blood pressure, leading to reduced peripheral skin temperature, making it harder to get to sleep<br>• Decreased water intake increases cardiac and sympathetic tone, which moves blood to the core, making it harder to cool at night, and harder to sleep |
| **Temperature** | • For sleep to occur, skin temperature must heat up as the core decreases<br>• The room temperature should be approximately 18°C but if the skin is cold, it becomes harder to transition into sleep – hence pyjamas and warms socks are important during winter for sleep!<br>• Taking a bath or shower before bed helps to warm the skin but cool the core, making the body ready for sleep |

linked to elevated levels of positive emotions, decreased negative emotions, and enhanced life satisfaction (Lenneis et al., 2024). This explains why, after a good night's sleep, we feel that life is good.

At the same time, each instance of sleep deprivation tends to diminish our experience of positive emotions, making them feel muted (Palmer et al., 2024). On such days, it can feel as though no matter how many positive experiences individuals encounter, they're unable to fully reap the benefits from them. Certain individuals, such as those with later chronotypes, may be particularly affected by the reduction in positive emotions during periods of sleep deprivation (Cox et al., 2024). Furthermore, our self-reported satisfaction with our sleep patterns holds significant weight. Some individuals may clock fewer hours of sleep yet still feel content with their rest, which can influence their overall subjective wellbeing (Lenneis et al., 2024). When we're content with the amount of sleep we're getting, our overall wellbeing tends to see an improvement.

Heart rate variability (HRV) plays an essential role in the relationship between sleep and positive emotions, as it amplifies the influence of quality sleep on positive emotions (Ballesio et al., 2023). HRV reflects the autonomic nervous system's regulation of heart rate and has been linked to overall health and wellbeing.

Individuals with favourable HRV patterns tend to experience greater benefits regarding positive emotional experiences after sleep. This suggests that HRV serves as a vital link between sleep and positive health outcomes. Conversely, those with unfavourable HRV may be more vulnerable to experiencing heightened anxiety or other negative emotions. Therefore, understanding the link between sleep and positive emotions and the factors influencing it is of utmost importance.

In addition to fleeting positive emotions, research has consistently linked meaning in life, life purpose, and sleep quality. For instance, individuals experiencing sleep disturbances, such as excessive or inadequate sleep, often reported lower levels of life purpose (Hamilton et al., 2007). However, those with a strong sense of purpose exhibited reduced body movement during sleep, leading to a marked improvement in sleep quality (Ryff et al., 2004). Furthermore, individuals with higher levels of self-reported purpose consistently reported better sleep outcomes, even after adjusting for demographic variables such as age and gender (Steptoe et al., 2009).

Importantly, purpose in life seems to act as a robust protective factor against developing sleep problems over time, potentially preventing sleep problems in the future (Phelan et al., 2010). As a sense of meaning in life is a cornerstone for overall wellbeing and physical health (Roepke et al., 2014; Steger, 2017), purpose and meaning in life can be a reliable source of comfort, ensuring individuals a good night's sleep.

Another aspect of eudaimonic wellbeing to consider is optimism, which numerous studies have correlated with sleep patterns. Optimism is crucial for resilience, enabling individuals to persevere through challenging circumstances. The opposite of optimism is a pessimistic outlook, which significantly elevates the risk of depression (Garrett & Sharot, 2017) and disrupts sleep quality (Uchino et al., 2017). In a cross-sectional study involving over 1,000 participants, optimistic individuals exhibited a notably reduced likelihood of experiencing insomnia compared to their pessimistic counterparts (Weitzer et al., 2021). In this study, optimism emerged as a more reliable predictor of sound sleep than lifestyle choices in this particular study.

Consequently, exploring interventions to foster a more optimistic mindset could hold promise for addressing insomnia. As outlined by Isaacowitz and Seligman (2002), cognitive behavioural therapy offers one such approach by assisting individuals in reshaping their thought patterns (Isaacowitz & Seligman, 2002). Health coaches specialising in positive psychology could also complement these efforts by helping patients identify and navigate between optimistic and pessimistic thinking patterns.

## COMMON SLEEP PROBLEMS

**Behaviourally Induced Insufficient Sleep Syndrome (BIIS)**. This voluntary restriction of sleep time is characterised by longer sleep duration at weekends and increased sleep debt (Abad & Guilleminault, 2003). BIIS impacts 7–20% of the general population, is common among 30–39-year-olds, those who abuse alcohol, experience chronic stress, are diagnosed with depression, and individuals who work more than 40 hours per week (Abad & Guilleminault, 2003).

**Chronic insomnia**. This sleep problem is characterised by difficulty initiating or maintaining sleep (frequent night or early waking). It occurs in the presence of adequate opportunity to sleep and is usually ongoing for three months, occurring at least three nights each week (Abad & Guilleminault, 2003). Chronic insomnia is commonly associated with co-occurring physical problems such as obesity, diagnosis with metabolic syndrome, high blood pressure, atrial fibrillation (irregular heartbeat), increased neck circumference and loud snoring. Cognitive Behavioural Therapy for Insomnia (CBT-I) is regarded as the gold standard treatment for insomnia (Walker et al., 2022).

**Obstructive sleep apnoea** is characterised by recurrent apnoea that lasts longer than ten seconds. Apnoea occurs when the muscles in the throat relax and collapse to block the airway (Punjabi, 2008). Up to 7% of adult men and 5% of adult women living in North America and Europe experience obstructive sleep apnoea at any given time (Punjabi, 2008). It is commonly associated with fatigue, malaise, sleepiness, poor concentration, memory impairment, poor judgement and errors, mood disturbance and irritability, headaches and gastrointestinal distress.

**Restless leg syndrome** is a sensorimotor condition associated with a strong urge to move limbs and torso when at rest (usually lower limbs, hence restless leg). It is sometimes associated with discomfort and pain, which worsens in the evenings. These symptoms are not due to another medical cause. Restless leg syndrome impacts 5–15% of the European population and is commonly associated with iron abnormalities (low serum ferritin <75 mg/dl) or high serum ferritin (Liu et al., 2022).

## SLEEP AND HEALTH

Common sense dictates that sleep is essential for health and wellbeing, which is supported in the scientific and medical literature. Adequate sleep enhances learning and memory, helps to manage emotional distress, increases cognitive processing speed, enhances fear extinguishing and emotional regulation, and has been shown to mitigate anxiety and depression (Scott et al., 2021).

We also know that sleep is essential for heart health (cardiovascular health). Sleep deficits lead to higher sympathetic tone (linked to adrenaline and fight or flight response), blood vessel injury, high blood lipids (fats), higher blood pressure at night, increased risk of heart attacks, and increased cardiovascular disease-related deaths (Berjaoui et al., 2023). Interestingly, US researchers noted increased numbers of individuals experiencing heart attacks that required life-saving surgery on the Monday following daylight savings changes in time during the spring (Sandhu et al., 2014). A corresponding reduction in heart attacks requiring surgery was observed in the autumn change (gain of an hour). This does not mean that losing or gaining an hour causes heart attacks. However, it does add to the data describing a link between adequate sleep and heart health.

Good sleep is commonly associated with deep NREM sleep and DNA repair, the routine production of anti-cancer cytokines, which are immune-related chemical messengers that include inter-leukin [IL]-1, IL-2, and Tumour Necrosis Factor [TNF]-α) (Berisha et al., 2022). Unfortunately, sleep has also been associated with several different cancers, such as those impacting the breast, endometrium, prostate cancer, rectum, and colon, as well as blood-borne cancers like acute myeloid leukaemia (Berisha et al., 2022). It remains unclear whether poor sleep and cancer development are causative or correlational.

### SLEEP HYGIENE TO PROMOTE HEALTHY SLEEP

Sleep hygiene encompasses practices supporting sleep while decreasing or eliminating those discouraging sleep (Irish et al., 2015). These behaviours cover everything from eliminating caffeine and alcohol to reducing carbohydrate-based food after 6 pm and avoiding blue light from mobile phones and other devices (Table 5.3). In addition to this, exploring some of the positive health interventions such as exploring meaning and purpose in life or improving optimism can also prove helpful in improving sleep (Burke et al., 2022). Poor sleep is linked to increased pessimism and decreased life satisfaction, while sufficient sleep enhances life satisfaction and reduces depression and anxiety. As described earlier in this section, cultivating meaning, purpose and optimism in life is important for adequate sleep.

*Table 5.3* Sleep hygiene practices include behaviours that when combined can support healthy sleep and help manage occasional insomnia

| *Sleep Hygiene Practice* |
| --- |
| Exercise in morning |
| At least 10-minute exposure to morning daylight |
| No large carbohydrate meals after 6 pm |
| Remove devices from bedroom |
| Hydrate in afternoon |
| Bath/shower before bed |
| Wake same time each morning including weekends |
| Avoid alcohol |
| Avoid caffeinated drinks after 12 noon |
| Bedroom is for sleep and sex only |

## POSITIVE PSYCHOLOGY INTERVENTIONS TO SUPPORT REGULAR HEALTHY SLEEP INCLUDE:

**Gratitude journaling**. Regularly writing down things for which one is grateful can help shift focus to positive aspects of life, thereby fostering a more optimistic outlook.

**Visualisation and mental pre-rehearsal of positive experiences**. Engaging in visualisation exercises where individuals imagine positive future outcomes can enhance optimism by creating a mental image of success and wellbeing.

**Strength-based exercises**. Identifying and using personal strengths in daily activities can boost confidence and foster an optimistic mindset (Littman-Ovadia et al., 2021).

**Meditation**. Practicing meditation (especially mindfulness-based incorporating non-judgemental awareness) can help individuals to become more aware of their thoughts and feelings, allowing them to redirect negative thoughts to more positive, optimistic ones.

**Cognitive behavioural techniques**. Techniques such as cognitive restructuring (re-framing) help individuals challenge and change negative thought patterns, promoting more optimistic thinking (Nakao et al., 2021).

**Practicing humour**. Prescribing laughter to university students based in the United Arab Emirates (UAE) improved health and wellbeing, including sleep quality and duration (Gonot-Schoupinsky et al., 2020).

## EATING HEALTHY FOOD

Many useful resources exist that provide examples of what a healthy food intake looks like. The healthy plate, produced by the Canadian government, provides a very useful illustration of this (Government of Canada, 2024). For a healthy plate: (1) make half your plate full of fresh fruit and vegetables (including leafy greens), (2) one quarter should be whole grains, and (3) the final quarter represents protein-based foods (dairy, eggs, meats and fish, beans, soy protein, nuts and peas). The final recommendation is to make water your drink of choice.

Unprocessed or minimally processed foods are close to their original state. They are usually only modified to preserve them by drying, roasting, boiling, or pasteurisation. Conversely, processed foods have added ingredients such as salt, oil, sugar, or other substances (like yeast and bicarbonate of soda in the case of bread). Common processed foods include canned fish, vegetables, fruits, and fresh bread. Finally, ultra-processed foods often contain added ingredients like sugar, salt, fat, and chemical additives. Ultra-processed food is made from refined, high-yielding foods (glucose syrup from sugar cane, gluten from wheat, soy from maize) and additives (artificial colours, flavours, and preservatives). Ultra-processed food includes frozen ready-meals, soft drinks, processed meats (sausages, bacon, hot dogs), fast food, crisps, and sweets (Leite et al., 2022). Ultra-processed food has a direct association with higher rates of heart disease, obesity, type 2 diabetes and mental health disorders (anxiety and depression) (Lane et al., 2024). Ultra-processed food accounts for 58% of all calories consumed by residents of the United States and 10% of the Italian diet (Lane et al., 2024).

*Table 5.4* Risky food intake and management

|  | *Recommendation* |
|---|---|
| **Salt** | A daily intake of 5g of salt, equivalent to 2g of sodium is recommended |
| **Free sugars** | Less than 10% of the daily diet (e.g., sugar added to tea and coffee) |
| **Industrially produced trans-fats (Omega 4, 5,6)** | It is best to avoid these fats, if possible |

## HEALTHY FOOD FOR A HEALTHY GUT

In a previous section, we discussed the importance of your gut microbiome to your physical and mental health. Prebiotic food is hugely important for maintaining the species that make up the gut microbiome and includes whole foods like fresh fruit and vegetables, seeds, nuts, beans, pulses, and whole grains that are all high in fibre. Furthermore, we know that eating fermented food containing these microorganisms and the fibre they like to eat (probiotic or symbiotic food) can also be an excellent way to keep their numbers topped up. However, this begs the question, what is fibre?

Fibre is found exclusively in plants and usually cannot be broken down in the human gut by digestive enzymes. However, probiotic species in the gut can break these complex sugars (oligosaccharides) into metabolites that have many health-related functions (Veronese et al., 2018). Fibre can be water soluble (found in peas, oats, barley, berries, and carrots, among other foods) or insoluble (potatoes, root vegetables, wheat, beans, cauliflower, wheat bran, nuts, etc.). Both types are essential for health, indicating that a varied diet is required here. Insoluble fibre is essential for transporting material through the gut. We know that fibre reduces mortality caused by cardiovascular disease (heart attacks and strokes).

## HEALTHY EATING IS MORE THAN ABOUT FOOD

The Canadian food guide (published by Health Canada) recommends: (1) be mindful as you shop; (2) be mindful as you eat (savour and be grateful); (3) try to cook your food more often; (4) cook and eat in the company of others, if you can; (5) use food labels to inform yourself; (6) avoid ultra-processed food; and (7) be aware of marketing designed to get you to eat unhealthy food (Health Canada, 2024).

## WHOLE FOOD PLANT-BASED DIETS AND NONCOMMUNICABLE DISEASE

The American College of lifestyle medicine uses several studies to showcase the power of whole food and plant-based diets to mitigate and, in some cases, reverse noncommunicable diseases such as uncontrolled high blood pressure, advanced cardiovascular disease, and type 2 diabetes.

### THE HARVARD NURSES' HEALTH STUDY (NHS)

This cohort study that began in 1976 has advanced our understanding of the risk factors associated with the development of non-communicable diseases (NCDs), especially cardiovascular disease and type 2 diabetes (Colditz et al., 2016). The NHS has enrolled over 120,000 registered nurses since 1976 and has collected extensive health data. The study has been vital in identifying the relationship between lifestyle factors and the risk of developing type 2 diabetes and cardiovascular diseases. Key findings include the association of smoking, diet, physical activity, and body weight with the risk of these diseases. Specifically, the study highlighted the preventative effect of a healthy diet and regular physical activity on NCDs. Study findings have demonstrated that up to 90% of type 2 diabetes cases could be prevented through appropriate health diet and lifestyle modifications.

### EPIC–OXFORD STUDY

The 1993 EPIC–Oxford study, part of the more extensive European Prospective Investigation into Cancer and Nutrition (EPIC), was a longitudinal study examining dietary impacts on health outcomes, including cardiovascular health and type 2 diabetes (Key et al., 2022). The study recruited 65,429 men and women (aged 20–97 years old) between 1993 and 1999. The study focused on the relationships between various dietary patterns, mainly vegetarian and non-vegetarian diets, and long-term health outcomes. It provided extensive data on how lifestyle choices, particularly diet, influence the prevalence and incidence of chronic diseases. The study suggests that plant-based diets are associated with a lower risk of developing cardiovascular diseases and type 2 diabetes. This aligns with evidence indicating that such diets reduce body mass index, cholesterol levels, and blood pressure, all risk factors for these conditions (Key et al., 2022). However, it should also be noted that vegan participants were at higher risk of developing ischaemic stroke. Plant-based diet participants also required supplementation to maintain health: vitamin B12, vitamin D, calcium, and iodine.

## A CAUTIONARY TALE FOR THOSE EATING A PREDOMINANTLY PLANT-BASED DIET

Sally is a 21-year-old university student. Most weeks involve at least four meat-free days. She is not a strict vegetarian, but values the predominantly plant-based diet. She feels so much better when she sticks to meat-free meals. After 12 months on this diet, Sally developed a tingling sensation in her hands and feet, often leading to partial numbness. She found this a little disturbing. Her doctor suspected that this numbness might be caused by a vitamin B12 deficiency. Blood tests confirmed that Sally was slightly deficient in vitamin B12. Sally subsequently receives regular injections with vitamin B12, which has solved the problem. This emphasises the point that vitamin B12 deficiency poses a real problem for many individuals on a partial vegetarian diet. Anyone embarking on this largely healthy journey should be vigilant in this regard. Interestingly, Sally also lives in a country where limited winter sunlight leads to vitamin D deficiency among the population. A plant-based diet free from dairy might exacerbate vitamin D deficiency. It is important to ask your GP to test the levels of important vitamins and minerals in your blood through testing on a frequent basis and proceed as an informed vegetarian.

### THE 7TH DAY ADVENTISTS HEALTH STUDY (AHS)

The 7th Day Adventists Health Study (AHS), a unique endeavour, was divided into two major studies. AHS-1 (n = 34,198) ran from 1974 to 1988, while AHS-2 began in 2002 (n = 96,000) and is still ongoing (Orlich et al., 2013). Both AHS studies delved into the links between lifestyle, diet, and disease among members of the 7th Day Adventist church, a Christian denomination primarily based in the city of Loma Linda (California, US). The study, one of the largest of its kind, specifically examines the benefits of whole food, predominantly plant-based diets on human health (Table 5.5).

### EATING WELL AND WELLBEING

Embracing a healthy diet is not just about physical health – it's a pathway to overall wellbeing. For example, following a

*Table 5.5* Key findings of the 7th Day Adventist Health Study, designed to examine the impact of whole food plant-based diet on health

| 7th Day Adventists Health Study | |
| --- | --- |
| **Fibre** | Vegetarians in the study had a lower risk than non-vegetarians for all cancers mentionedVegetarians were less obese, consumed less coffee, exercised more regularly, and ate more legumes and vegetarian protein products |
| **Fruit** | Eating fruit twice daily had a 75% risk reduction in cancer compared with those who ate fruit less than three times a week for lung cancer risk |
| **Legumes (beans, lentils, and peas)** | Individuals who eat beans at least twice a week had a 42% lower risk of colon cancer than those who ate beans less than once a week. Eating legumes more than three times a week had a 47% lower risk of prostate cancer, while those eating legumes more than twice a week had a much lower risk of pancreatic cancer |
| **Red meat** | Consuming beef may increase the risk of fatal coronary heart disease for men; Adventist men who ate beef more than twice a week experienced a significant increase in fatal coronary heart disease. Beef consumption did not alter the risk of heart disease in women |
| **Whole-wheat bread** | Eating whole-wheat bread can protect against heart disease. Consuming mainly whole-wheat bread had a relative risk of 59% for nonfatal CHD and 89% for fatal heart disease compared to those who ate a standard Western diet |
| **Nuts** | Nut consumption reduced the risk of both fatal and nonfatal CHD |

Mediterranean diet enhances both health and subjective wellbeing (Moreno-Agostino et al., 2019). In blue zones, where people's health thrives, their communities also enjoy high levels of mental wellbeing (Buettner & Skemp, 2016; Hitchcott et al., 2018). This evidence suggests a strong association between what we eat and our mental health.

However, healthy eating is not just about following diets; iwhot is also about enhancing your wellbeing by increasing your intake of fruits and vegetables. Research by Mujcic and Oswald (2016) has shown that higher consumption of fruits and vegetables is associated with increased happiness, life satisfaction, and overall wellbeing. Additionally, consuming fruits and vegetables predicts higher positive emotions (Warner et al., 2017). According to two studies, at least 7–8 servings of fruits or vegetables daily are necessary to see meaningful changes (Blanchflower et al., 2013; Mujcic & Oswald, 2016). These changes include feeling calmer, happier, and more energetic, with the positive mood often lasting into the next day. Therefore, combining lifestyle and wellbeing interventions can be a powerful tool for achieving positive health benefits. Research also shows that keeping a diary of your fruit and vegetable consumption for two weeks can lead to greater emotional wellbeing and higher levels of curiosity and creativity (Conner et al., 2015).

### POSITIVE PSYCHOLOGY INTERVENTIONS TO SUPPORT REGULAR PHYSICAL ACTIVITY AND EXERCISE

The most researched and evidence-based Positive Psychology Interventions (Burke et al., 2022) to support healthy eating include:

- **Gratitude practice**. Expressing gratitude for the food available in your locality and the ability to nourish one's body can enhance a positive relationship with food and encourage mindful eating (Fritz et al., 2019). Be grateful for the hands that grew and prepared the food. Sense the immense connection to other people through your food.
- **Mindful eating**. Practising mindfulness while preparing, cooking, as well as during meals, such as paying attention to the taste, texture, and aroma of food, can reduce overeating, enhance enjoyment of food, and promote healthier eating patterns (Khan & Zadeh, 2014).
- **Social Support**. Engaging with a supportive community or network, such as joining a healthy eating group or sharing goals with friends and family, can provide encouragement, accountability, and shared experiences that promote healthier eating habits. Above all else, research shows (Glanz et al., 2021) that eating regular healthy meals with others promotes health and wellbeing.

## A FINAL WORD ON FOOD

Although general guidelines exist on consuming healthy food, and we know that eating large amounts of ultra-processed foods is bad for our health, there is still no one-size-fits-all approach. One person's joy in eating brussels sprouts represents hell for another. Assuming balance and common sense, I believe that American Journalist Michael Pollan said it all when he wrote: "Eat food. Not too much. Mostly plants" (Pollan, 2009).

## PHYSICAL ACTIVITY

Physical activity involves any bodily movement produced by skeletal muscles that requires energy expenditure. Exercise, on the other hand, is a subcategory of physical activity that is planned, structured, repetitive, and purposeful; the objective of exercise is to improve or maintain one or more components of physical fitness. Fitness measures the body's ability to function efficiently and effectively in work and leisure activities; it includes physical and cardiorespiratory fitness. Physical fitness encompasses five essential elements for whole health: cardiorespiratory endurance, muscle strength, muscle endurance, body composition, and flexibility (WHO, 2022).

## METABOLIC EQUIVALENT OF TASK (MET)

Healthcare professionals sometimes measure energy expenditure and sedentary behaviour as METs, a physiological measure expressing the intensity of physical activities. One MET is the energy equivalent an individual spends while seated at rest. One of the biggest threats to physical fitness in the 21st century is sedentary behaviour, defined as any waking behaviour characterised by an energy expenditure of 1.5 METS or lower while sitting, reclining, or lying. Most desk-based office work, driving a car, and watching television are examples of sedentary behaviours; these can also apply to those unable to stand, such as wheelchair users. The recommended guidelines for exercise for all age groups are presented in Table 5.6.

## THE COMPONENTS OF EXERCISE

We can have many goals when we exercise depending on our needs, age, gender, and health status. In general, the components of

*Table 5.6* Recommended exercise guidelines for exercise (WHO, 2020)

| Demographic | Aerobic | Strength | Flexibility & balance |
| --- | --- | --- | --- |
| **Children and adolescents** (5–17 years) | 60 minutes of moderate to vigorous intensity daily | 3 days each week strengthening bodies and engaging in vigorous aerobic exercise | |
| **Adults** (18–64 years) | 150–300 minutes of moderate intensity each week | 2 days each week of moderate intensity, working on all muscle groups | |
| **Older adults** (65 years and older) | 150–300 minutes of moderate intensity each week | 2 days each week of moderate intensity, working on all muscle groups | 3 days each week, engage in multi-component exercise that includes balance and flexibility with strength and aerobic |

exercise include agility (the capacity to move the body with speed, in different directions with accuracy), balance, body composition (percentage of fat, bone, muscle, and other tissues within the body), cardiorespiratory fitness (the ability of the heart and lungs to supply oxygen during exercise), coordination, flexibility (range of mobility in any joint), muscular endurance and strength, power, reaction time, and speed (Farley et al., 2020).

> **Moderate versus vigorous intensity – how can you tell?**
> Imagine you are out exercising with a friend at a local park. You are exercising at "moderate intensity" when you can talk to your friend but not sing the intro to your favourite musical. You are exercising at "vigorous intensity" when you can neither talk nor sing to your friend.

## EXERCISE AS MEDICINE

Regular physical exercise has been shown to exert a significant positive impact (Table 5.7) on promoting mental and physical health

*Table 5.7* Impact of regular exercise on different health parameters among different age groups

| Age group | Impact on health |
| --- | --- |
| **3 to <6 years** | Improved bone health and weight |
| **6 to 17 years** | Improved cognitive function |
| **Adult** | Lower incidents of heart disease, high blood pressure, and type 2 diabetes |
| | Lower incidence of bladder, breast, colon, endometrial, oesophageal, kidney, stomach, and lung cancers |
| | Reduced risk of dementia, depression, and anxiety |
| | Improved sleep and quality of life |
| | Reduced excessive weight gain |

Source: Piercy et al. (2018).

while also reducing the risk of developing common NCDs and certain cancers (Misiąg et al., 2022; Piercy et al., 2018).

## EXERCISE PRESCRIPTIONS USING THE FREQUENCY–INTENSITY–TIME–TYPE (FITT) PRINCIPLE

The FITT principle is a beneficial way to organise an exercise plan (Table 5.8) that can lead to sustained adherence to plans and improved health outcomes (Bland et al., 2021).

## CONSCIOUS EXERCISE AND MINDSET

What if your household chores could be viewed as part of your planned weekly exercise? Why not get some health benefits from those daily and weekly annoyances? In a 2007 study, Crum and co-workers conducted a controlled study with 84 female room attendants based at seven hotels in Manhattan, New York. They wanted to test the impact of mindset on the relationship between exercise and health (Crum & Langer, 2007). Before the four-week study, all participants were measured for baseline weight, body mass index (BMI), blood pressure, body fat, and waist-to-hip ratio. The intervention group participants were educated on the recommended weekly exercise guidelines and asked to view their daily

*Table 5.8* Exercise prescription using the FITT framework

| FITT | Impact on health | Example based on WHO guidelines for strength training among adults |
|------|------------------|---------------------------------------------------------------------|
| **Frequency** | The number of times the exercise is repeated | 3 days each week with a rest day in-between |
| **Intensity** | The difficulty level | Moderate |
| **Time** | Duration | 20 minutes per session |
| **Type** | The type of exercise (weights, squats etc.) | Squats with 7.5 Kg weights in each hand, over 25 M (× 2 REPS; repetitions)Plank for 30 seconds with 10 second rest (× 3 REPS) Hold press-up for 30 seconds with 10 second rest (× 3 REPS) Wall squats for 30 seconds with 10 second rest (× 3 REPS) |

Source: Piercy et al. (2018).

work as part of an exercise routine. The control group were asked to work as usual. Four weeks later, intervention group participants had significantly improved health outcomes with decreased weight, blood pressure, body fat, waist-to-hip ratio, and BMI compared to their control counterparts (Crum & Langer, 2007). Therefore, how we perceive physical activity (e.g., household chores) can improve health outcomes.

## COMMUNITY-BASED EXERCISE VERSUS EXERCISING ALONE

Cultivating positive relationships is a pillar of lifestyle medicine. Therefore, exercising in a community (or group) context positively impacts health more than exercising alone.

## LESSONS FROM PARKRUN IN THE UK

The Parkrun is an ever-increasing global phenomenon where citizens can run (or walk) at free, weekly, 5km and 2km community events in open spaces within their locality. Scientists in the United Kingdom tested a hypothesis that people engaging in Parkruns in groups would benefit more physically and psychosocially than those who ran alone. One hundred and forty-three Parkrun participants, running at six

Parkrun sites in southern England, were surveyed multiple times in 2015. The subsequent study findings revealed that social reward and community-based support in exercise were associated with positive self-reported exercise experiences (greater subjective enjoyment and less fatigue) and greater performance outcomes (faster run times) than individuals who ran alone (Davis et al., 2021).

## GROUP EXERCISE TO PREVENT COGNITIVE DECLINE

Japanese citizens (n=4,358; mean age=76; 51.8% female) completed a nationally standardised dementia scale by mail in 2017 and were asked about their exercise routines. The same individuals were followed until 2021 and regularly surveyed for cognitive impairment. Those citizens who exercised in groups showed a 29.2% decreased risk of dementia and cognitive decline compared with those who exercised alone or not at all (Nagata et al., 2023).

## POSITIVE PSYCHOLOGY INTERVENTIONS TO SUPPORT REGULAR PHYSICAL ACTIVITY AND EXERCISE

The most researched positive psychology tools (Burke et al., 2022) to support physical exercise include:

- **Cultivating a growth mindset**. Failure is a regular consequence of human engagement and practices (Dweck & Yeager, 2019). It is normal and depending on your mindset can either offer a wonderful opportunity to learn or reflects deficiency and a sense of inadequacy. Cultivate the former.
- **Developing and sustaining a sense of self-compassion**. Physical activity and exercise in particular can be difficult to sustain. Cultivate regular self-compassion-based practices such as loving-kindness meditation or journal about the nature of compassion. Challenge the inner critic through cognitive behavioural approaches or via attention-based training (ABT) techniques (Dunne et al., 2019).
- **Cultivating social support**. Engaging with a community, such as joining a fitness group or having an exercise buddy, can provide encouragement, accountability, and a sense of belonging, which promotes consistent exercise habits (Davis et al., 2021).

**Positive reinforcement**. Rewarding oneself for meeting exercise milestones or achieving goals can reinforce the behaviour and create a positive association with physical activity.

**Visualisation and mental pre-rehearsal**. Imagining the successful completion of exercise goals and visualising the benefits of physical activity can enhance motivation and performance.

**Gratitude practice**. Expressing gratitude for one's physical abilities and health can foster a positive mindset towards exercise and encourage regular physical activity.

**Meditation**. Practising meditation can help individuals focus on the present moment (conscious exercise), and enhance the overall exercise experience, making it more enjoyable and sustainable in the long run (Edwards & Loprinzi, 2018).

Encouraging humans to engage in physical activity and exercise as a means to better health and longer health span is complex with no straightforward one-size-fits-all approach. As humans, we come in all shapes and sizes with different capacities for different exercises, depending on a dizzying array of modifying parameters. Exercising alone is excellent for some but so much for others. However, one thing that is clear is that some kind of exercise each day is necessary for health. Exercise might be used as a medicine by itself and, in some cases, help reverse NCD development and even support recovery from certain cancers. Find what type of exercise you can fall in love with and do it (as someone once said). Whether walking the dogs, kayaking, biking to work, or washing your windows at home, it is all good as long as you do it.

### Liam's story

*Liam is a male 68-year-old retiree. He retired from 42 years in the same sheet metal factory that his Dad and uncle attended. Liam is conservative in outlook and mindset. He believes that men should be men and is not enamoured with what he sees as woke society. He feels that the world has taken a turn for the worst. Liam had a difficult childhood, where he was exposed to several forms of abuse from the Christian Brothers who ran his local primary school. This is one of the reasons why he left school at 14 to join his father and uncle in the work place. He has always had a lingering sense of inadequacy that is protected by a gruff and occasionally rude exterior. He has rarely spoken about his childhood and has a difficult relationship with his two daughters and ex-wife.*

*Liam lives alone with his Jack Russel dog (Ned). Since retiring, he has become morbidly obese with a BMI of 39, high (uncontrolled) blood pressure and is pre-diabetic, according to recent blood sugar and HbA1c assessments. During his most recent visit to his doctor, he was informed that he is unlikely to reach the age of 70 if he continues with his lifestyle.*

*This is the first time that he has considered his own mortality – his father died at 63 but he was a heavy smoker; Liam doesn't smoke. The doctor's message has shaken him but he's not sure where to turn. His neighbour is a member of a local Men's Shed group but he is reluctant to join them. Two of his old school mates go there and he doesn't like them very much. He tentatively asks his neighbour over the back fence about the Men's Shed group and what the meetings entail.*

*After much soul searching, he decides to go and although he was extremely nervous and didn't say a thing to anyone for the two hours he was there, he did feel better when he got home. Some weeks later, he was asked to give advice on how to weld garden structures from old scrap metal by the nominal leader of the Men's Shed group. Although he got frustrated sometimes with some of the men, he enjoyed this – he never thought he would be a teacher of any kind.*

*Liam hasn't changed his eating habits much and he is still over-weight but he feels a little better about his life. He still doesn't like a lot of the men who attend the Men's Shed but some of them are alright. He decided to make walking early in the morning along the new ring-road, a regular occurrence. He was surprised that this helped a little with his sleep and his dog Ned has lost some weight. He thinks that if there's hope for Ned, there might be hope for him. Time will tell but he feels a little less pessimistic about life and people.*

## STRESS MANAGEMENT

We described the biology of stress in Chapter 4 and noted that not all stress is bad; stress can be quite helpful and help prepare us to compete, achieve, and evolve as humans. Our stress responses have not changed in thousands of years, something we share with our mammalian friends. We also know that humans add an extra layer of complexity to the stress response through our capacity to think about past events and worry about future potentials. This is captured perfectly in Robert Sapolsky's book, *Why Zebras Don't Get Ulcers* (Sapolsky, 2004). Although not as powerful, in terms of a physiological response, a perceived internal threat will create a chain reaction, resulting in activation of the HPA axis, adrenaline, and cortisol production. In the long term, this leads to a dysfunctional immune response, altered metabolism (fatigue, weight loss, or weight gain), anhedonia (an urge to retire to your bedroom and stay away from everything), and sometimes intermittent bouts of panic, fear, and anxiety leading to depression. This physiological and psychological response to internal or external threats can be seen as typical. Even though we might always be able to avoid stressors (loss of a job, illness, exam-related pressure), we can certainly learn how to manage our response to them.

Much of this book is dedicated to positive psychology theory and interventions designed to lift a human from a functioning state into a flourishing or thriving one. These evidence-based approaches naturally dovetail with what I will discuss below. The best way to deal with stress is to accept that it is an inevitable part of every human life and prepare for it by engaging in daily positive health-related practices. This approach is not magic and will not stave off life's difficulties. However, it will serve as a buffer to help you manage these eventualities.

### AWARENESS

Step one is to enhance your awareness of your internal thinking processes, how you view your world (inside and out), your body and how it feels, and your sense of place in the world as a human being. After all, if you are unaware of the problem, how can you develop a strategy to manage it?

You can start with validated psychological surveys (Positive Psychology Center, 2024) that can help you identify emerging issues. Although positive psychology moves away from a deficit approach to wellbeing to focus on strengths, gratitude, and optimism, sometimes it is important to note a rising inner critic that can be largely subconscious or tightening back muscles over time. For example, you can test your levels of burnout using the Maslach Burnout Inventory

(Maslach & Jackson, 1981). Burnout can be insidious; it can sneak up on you without notice.

Journaling can be a magnificent and safe way to unveil and enhance awareness of your thoughts, emotions, and emerging memories (Burke et al., 2022). It can also be an excellent way to show you your progress. Sometimes, we feel like we are going nowhere, but a journal can show you this progress in black and white as you flip back through the pages. Journaling can have a focus (gratitude, for example); however, to enhance awareness, we take the shackles off and let whatever comes to the page come.

Speaking with other safe human beings can be a constructive way to enhance self-awareness. By telling our stories to others, we often see a reflection of ourselves that was hitherto unknown; we can see blind spots. Of course, one of the best ways to do this is to speak with a counsellor or psychotherapist who can help you unpack your thoughts, emotions and memories in a way that can be safe but also very revealing. We do not have to have a mental health problem to seek support from a counsellor or psychotherapist. Engaging a health professional can stave off mental health issues and stress by enhancing awareness of self regularly.

Meditation tools can also be beneficial in enhancing awareness. Mindfulness meditation has emerged as one of the most researched meditation practices (Creswell, 2017). It involves observing thoughts, emotions, sensations, and memories in a non-reactive, non-judgemental way. Sometimes referred to as insight meditation (alluding to its Buddhist origins), this practice can help us reveal our inner processes, which, on occasion, might involve distorted opinions and assumptions about the self and others. It can reveal loves, fears, and authentic interests. The body scan is another practice that creates awareness of what is happening in the body. We frequently ignore the body and act like a giant head riding on a little donkey. We only notice the donkey when it is in pain or discomfort or when it doesn't look like other donkeys. Hopefully, it will have become apparent through the contents of this book that all our psychological, physical, and social systems are intertwined; what impacts one will impact the other, for good or bad. Paying regular attention to the body can help us see muscle tension development. We can use the body scan meditation to guide us to these hot spots, where we can stop and consciously relax the area. It is also helpful to help calm the body when stressed, angry, frustrated, or upset before engaging in meditative practice. The body scan can also be helpful when you wake between 2 and 4 am and find it hard to get back to sleep. Once you get used to the guided practice, you try guiding yourself through the process, which means you are not dependent on a phone or Wi-Fi connection to access it.

As with all wellbeing practices, there is no one-size-fits-all, and not everyone can sit in silence and engage in this type of practice, at least not easily. It is also advised that anyone with severe trauma (especially recent trauma) should see support from a psychotherapist prior to engaging in meditation practices for safety.

You can create an awareness of aspects of lifestyle medicine practice that require attention by completing one of two suggested surveys (dependent on your needs). The first is the US Department of Veterans Affairs, Personal Health Inventory (PHI), which offers a chance to score yourself in areas such as relaxation/healing time, the health of your environment, energy and flexibility, human connections, family and co-workers, sleep, health food, exercise, and personal development (US Department of Veterans Affairs, 2022). This self-reported questionnaire involves completing simple Likert scale questions on the above items. It is not a diagnostic test but can help you identify areas of unmet need. An equivalent questionnaire that requires more detail regarding the pillars of lifestyle medicine is the Lifestyle Assessment Long Form, which is also very useful (Loma Linda University, 2024). This assessment was created between the American College of lifestyle medicine and Loma Linda University of Health.

## THE IMPORTANCE OF BREATHING

The breath has been posited as a gateway to health for thousands of years, and many religions and cultures have advocated different practices. There are many different types of breathing techniques, many of which have some evidence of being able to boost health outcomes, including those related to mental health (McKeown, 2021). We know that the US Military advise box-breathing (inhale for 5 seconds – hold for 5 – exhale for 5 – hold for five, etc.) (Divine, 2016). We also know that professional athletes use it to reset their minds and body before engaging on the field (Dymock, 2024).

Slow-paced breathing practices are the most researched, and there are several supporting theories on how they might work. One supporting theory is related to respiratory sinus arrhythmia (RSA), whereby when we breathe, our heart rate increases (imperceptibly), which is associated with the sympathetic arm of the ANS (see Chapter 4) (Yasuma & Hayano, 2004). Conversely, when we exhale, our heart rate reduces, linked to the parasympathetic arm of the ANS, particularly the vagus nerve. Stress is often associated with shallow breathing that is over-focused on inhalation, interrupted by occasional sighing (deep inhalation, followed by extended exhalation (Balban et al., 2023).

Fincham and colleagues in the United Kingdom conducted a 2023 meta-analysis (a report of published studies) of 12 research projects designed to investigate breathing as an intervention to mitigate stress (Fincham et al., 2023). After examining these studies (785 participants), Fincham and co-workers report that breathing techniques mitigated stress more than control groups (medium effect size). However, they caution that many studies show a degree of bias, which requires more robust, less heterogeneous future research.

Although the jury is still out (in terms of research), breathing is an effective way to manage physical stress in the body and serves to calm the mind. It would seem that equalising inhalation with exhalation, either through tactical box breathing or simply counting for 5 seconds in and 5 seconds out, can restore balance to the ANS. Likewise, extending the exhalation and thereby indirectly activating the parasympathetic nerves (e.g., 4-7-8 breathing) might help to calm you when agitated, angry, or upset.

## MEDITATION

Between 2000 and April 2024, the PubMed database listed 9,235 research articles and reviews mentioning "meditation" in titles or abstracts. While not all are top-quality, the volume underscores the field's rapid growth, attracting researchers from neuroscience, medicine, psychology, behavioural science, sociology, and more.

Studying meditation's effects is challenging compared to drug trials. Double-blind, randomised controlled trials work well for pharmacological agents but are impractical for meditation, where blinding is impossible. The Hawthorne Effect (McCambridge et al., 2014) and often low participant numbers pose additional challenges, resulting in studies with small samples aware of their treatment, diminishing the power compared to pharmacological trials.

Despite these difficulties, rigorous global research consistently shows meditation's benefits on mental health, particularly with anxiety, stress, and burnout, and extends to pain, immune, hormone, and cardiovascular systems (Creswell, 2017; Dunne et al., 2019; Gawrylewski, 2018; Ridge et al., 2021). Exciting evidence also suggests the potential epigenetic impacts of meditation practice (Kaliman, 2019; Kaliman et al., 2014).

---

### DIFFERENT MEDITATION TYPES HAVE DIFFERENT BENEFITS

- Metacognition (like mindfulness)
- Concentration-based practices (e.g., Attention-based Training (ABT), mantra, Zazen)
- Compassion/gratitude-focused methods (like loving-kindness meditation)

---

The Max Planck Neuroscience Lab's ReSource Project further validated this by showing the distinct impacts of these practices on the brain, body, and behaviour (Singer & Engert, 2019). For personal practice, starting with a basic posture and a 2-minute focus on breathing or a mantra helps build concentration. Persistence and gradual extension of practice time can turn meditation into a habit within 66 days (Lally et al., 2010). You can find several meditation-based resources, including our free ABT programme, on our RCSI website.

#### BUILDING YOUR THRIVING TOOLKIT

As individuals, we respond differently to stimuli and practices depending on our stage of life, gender, cultural background, profession, etc. We suggest building a thriving toolkit to help you manage stress from several theoretical bases, including the interventions suggested in this book and having at least one grounding technique that places you in the present moment. That can be engaging in nature, with animals or other trusted humans, meditating, practising breathwork, playing music, writing, art, including theatre, and singing (Burke et al., 2022). Connecting to the mind, body, social and physical environment will help stay present; we know that a persistently wandering mind is generally unhappy (Killingsworth & Gilbert, 2010). Try to cultivate positive relationships with other humans and in your community. Stay calm if you do not have close family members or a partner. Research from Fredrickson has shown us that we can make strong, health-promoting human connections with non-family members and loved ones (Fredrickson et al., 2008).

Cultivating the body through lifestyle medicine's pillars is another essential part of any thriving toolkit that mitigates inevitable stress. This includes adequate sleep, eating healthy food, including prebiotics, daily physical activity (preferably outside in nature, if you can), and involvement in your community (if you can).

Finally, the capstone for any stress-mitigating thriving toolkit is cultivating self-compassion and a growth mindset. We know from the work of Carol Dweck that failures are inevitable, teaching moments for every human being (Dweck & Yeager, 2019). If we can view these failures as opportunities to learn and grow, we will have a growth mindset that will help during stressful times. We can learn to boycott the inner critic and cultivate compassion through meditation practices like loving-kindness and gratitude. Be gentle with yourself but persist with the journey.

### Anna's story

*Anna is a 15-year old Ukrainian female who has been displaced along with her mother by the war with Russia. The early days of the war in Kiev were fraught with tension, anxiety, and the threat of waking up to bombs and missiles that could kill her and her family at any moment. The dark nights were the worst. She spent days in state of heightened fear without much sleep. Her father and grandfather decided to stay in their family apartment but wanted Anna and her mother to move to a safe European country that spoke English – both Anna and her mother speak a little but are not fluent. They reluctantly left their family and home three months after the invasion.*

Unfortunately, Anna brought the fear, anxiety, and worry with her. Anna and her mother were re-housed in a hotel during the winter in a quiet seaside town. It's strange and a little bleak but at least it's safe. The kids in her new school are nice, as are the teachers, but it is hard to make friends and be open for her, even at the best of times.

She is seriously underweight and sleeps very little, which means she is always tired and has little energy. She feels on edge all the time. The smallest bang or rattle from a passing car, kids shouting, or a loud TV, seem to electrocute her. She has become irritable with her mother and hates that; she loves her mother and knows that it is hard for both of them.

Her music teacher asks Anna if she would like to join a choir after school. She's not sure but her mother thinks it might be good for her. The kids can choose some of the songs while the teacher picks the rest. Her teacher explains the importance of controlled breathing when singing, so that she doesn't get out of breath. It seems a little awkward at first (socially and physically) but after a month, she simply couldn't do without it. There is something about the social connection, the practice, and the act of singing in the moment that makes everything negative move to the periphery. When she sings, she experiences a focus and calm that she has never experienced before, even before the war. Singing opens doors for Anna. She has started two new ventures since joining the choir.

First, she decided to create a gratitude journal on a weekly basis on her phone. She saw an American teenager talk about it on TikTok and although initially sceptical, she gave it a try. It seemed strange at first; what had she to be grateful for? Apart form her mother, everyone she loved was in Ukraine. Her homeland was invaded by a brutal army and she had left most her material possessions behind. After some time, she realised that she was grateful for several things, in spite of her suffering and that of her family and country. This was not going to magically go away. However, she was grateful for being alive and for the support she received in her adopted country.

Second, she decided to talk to a local Ukrainian counsellor about her fear and anxiety. This has helped but she knows it will be a long journey. She is feeling a little better but longs to return home to a peaceful country.

# AVOIDING RISKY SUBSTANCES

**ALCOHOL**

## *What Is a Standard Drink?*

A standard drink is a measure of alcohol. In Ireland, one standard drink contains 10 grams of pure alcohol. Common examples include a half pint of 4.5% lager, a 100 ml glass of 12.5% wine and one pub measure of 40% spirits. The number of standard drinks is based on the size of the drink and its alcohol strength, usually shown on labels as alcohol by volume (% ABV). The higher the alcohol strength, the higher the standard drink content (Drinkaware, 2024).

## *Low-risk Guidelines*

- **Women**: Fewer than 11 standard drinks (110g pure alcohol) spread out over the week, with at least two alcohol-free days. E.g., <11 glasses of wine; 5 pints of 4.5% lager; <11 pub measures of 40% spirits.
- **Men**: Fewer than 17 standard drinks (170g pure alcohol) spread out over the week, with at least two alcohol-free days. E.g., <17 glasses of wine; 8 pints of 4.5 % lager; <17 pub measures of 40% spirits.

It takes your body one hour to process one standard drink. However, this should be taken as a guide for information purposes only. Many factors will affect this time, including age, gender, weight, alcohol strength, the speed of your metabolism, and the number of drinks consumed. Binge drinking is associated with causing harm and involves consuming six or more standard drinks in one sitting (Drinkaware, 2024).

The harm that long-term alcohol consumption can exert on the psychological, physical and social health of a person is long and well-documented (Iranpour & Nakhaee, 2019). Drinking alcohol can contribute to the development of cancers (breast, oral, and colon cancers), cardiovascular disease and high blood pressure, infectious diseases like tuberculosis, liver cirrhosis, suicides, as well as interpersonal conflict and violence (including domestic violence). Anyone worried about alcohol consumption should visit their local health-care provider.

## TOBACCO SMOKING AND E-CIGARETTES

It is now a well-established fact that smoking tobacco severely impacts health, causing lung cancer, chronic obstructive lung disease (COPD), cardiovascular disease, recurrent infections, and issues with fertility and pregnancy (Le Foll et al., 2022; West, 2017). However, many may not be aware of the negative impacts of second-hand smoke. Smokers only inhale a small percentage (approximately 15%) of the smoke from a cigarette; the remainder goes into the local environment or is inhaled by adjacent individuals (Health, 2024). Second-hand smoke contains carcinogens, which have been reported to make co-habitants 27% more likely to get lung cancer (HSE, 2024). Co-habiting children are also impacted by second-hand smoke, with an increased incidence of ear infections, asthma, allergies, meningitis, cancer, bronchitis, and pneumonia compared with children who live in smoking-free households (HSE, 2024). In addition, children who grow up seeing their parents smoke are three times more likely to smoke in adulthood (HSE, 2024). However, the good news is that the body can recover once smoking tobacco has ceased (Table 5.9). After just 72 hours, breathing improves and energy levels increase (HSE, 2024).

*Table 5.9* The positive impacts of quitting smoking on the body over time

| *What happens when you stop?* | |
| --- | --- |
| **20 minutes** | Your circulation improves; your blood pressure and heart rate get lower; your risk of a heart attack starts to reduce |
| **8 hours** | The nicotine and carbon monoxide levels in your blood go down and the oxygen level rises |
| **48 hours** | The nicotine and carbon monoxide leave your body; your sense of smell and taste starts to improve |
| **72 hours** | Your breathing improves and your energy levels increase |
| **3 months** | Your lung capacity will increase by up to 30% |
| **1 year** | Your chance of having a heart attack drops by half |
| **5 years** | The risk of smoking-related cancers is greatly reduced |
| **10 years** | The risk of lung cancer is reduced by half |

## E-cigarettes

E-cigarettes are often considered safer than conventional cigarettes since they don't involve tobacco combustion; instead, an internal battery heats the e-liquid, producing a vapour. However, this claim remains contentious due to the limited evidence available and the potential risks associated with their use. The process of heating e-liquid can create new compounds with known toxicity, such as acetaldehyde, formaldehyde, propylene oxide, and acrolein (Marques et al., 2021). Studies suggest that while e-cigarettes might be less hazardous than traditional cigarettes, they still pose health risks (Marques et al., 2021). Moreover, the long-term effects of e-cigarettes need to be better understood. They are under-researched, making it difficult to endorse their safety fully. The use of e-cigarettes also raises concerns regarding their role in smoking cessation and their impact during respiratory illnesses like COVID-19. Thus, while e-cigarettes offer a smoke-free alternative, their safety profile could be more benign, and more research is needed to understand their health implications fully.

### SOLUTIONS TO QUITTING SMOKING

Pharmacotherapy (medication-based therapy) that supports individuals to quit includes over-the-counter nicotine replacement therapy (e.g., gum and lozenges) and prescription medication such as Varenicline (nicotine receptor partial agonist) and Bupropion (noradrenaline/dopamine re-uptake inhibitor) (HSE, 2024). Although less harmful than cigarettes, e-cigarettes are not harm-free and, therefore, not recommended as part of a support system for smokers who wish to stop.

Furthermore, in the context of positive health, various interventions leveraging positive psychology have been developed to assist smokers in quitting. For instance, Harvard researchers created a smartphone application (app) called *Smiling Instead of Smoking*, designed to support non-daily smokers in quitting (Hoeppner et al., 2017). This smartphone app, which is grounded in the principles of positive psychology, includes interventions such as enlisting social support, or practising positive psychology interventions throughout the day. Results indicated that the app was effective for most participants, with 87% successfully quitting smoking and 82% maintaining a positive outlook during the process (Hoeppner et al., 2021). This research highlighted the advantages of prioritising wellbeing alongside promoting a healthy lifestyle. However, more research is needed to investigate whether this approach is impactful for heavy smokers. The optimal treatment plan for quitting smoking permanently still involves a combination of behavioural therapy and support, plus nicotine replacement therapy (e.g., patches or lozenges).

Best practice in terms of treatment still shows that behavioural, and nicotine replacement therapy is the effective thus far at supporting individuals to quit smoking permanently. Hopefully, positive health interventions can be added to this approach in the future.

### SMOKING AND WELLBEING

Smoking is associated with lower levels of wellbeing (Stanisławska Kubiak et al., 2019). In this study of 552 medical sciences students based in Poznań (Poland), researchers learned that smokers experienced more negative emotions, were less likely to experience pleasant emotions and felt more frustrated, compared to non-smokers and former smokers. Additionally, smokers examined in this study were less interested, inspired, attentive, determined, and active, compared to former smokers surveyed from the same University (Stanisławska Kubiak et al., 2019).

## SUMMARY

Humans do not exist in isolation. We coexist in complex, interdependent environments with other humans, animals, plants, and microbiomes. The microbiomes that coexist within and on human beings are responsible for healthy function and survival. Likewise, the social, political, fiscal, and physical environments also contribute to the health and wellbeing of each human. Loneliness, social isolation, and dysfunction, poverty, environmental pollution, and oppressive and corrupt government encompass the social determinants of human health.

Since the Enlightenment of the 18th century, scientists and healthcare professionals have endeavoured to establish the workings of the human mind, brain, and body using a reductionist approach.

The human body and mind were viewed as a mechanism that, once taken apart, would reveal their function and purpose. The complexity of human biology and psychology meant that scientists specialised in different fields of study; this saw the birth of scientific and medical subjects like psychology, cardiology, pathology, and surgery. Humans find it easier to understand complex processes by dividing them first into categories. The result was a logarithmic explosion in scientific discovery, cures for most infectious diseases, and medicines to prevent and treat many illnesses; countless millions have been saved and kept alive. Unfortunately, one of the consequences of this specialisation in healthcare and medicine was the assumption and false perception that our minds, bodies, and social environments are disconnected, self-determining units. For much of the 20th century, the idea that your mood or mental health status could impact your physiology was not considered.

We now know that our thinking processes, emotional reactions, and internal perceptions can have a direct impact (often within seconds) on our peripheral nervous system, our immune and endocrine systems, and the expression of our DNA. It is clear from emerging research that early adverse childhood experiences can exert a profoundly negative effect on all of these systems, leading to serious behavioural, psychological, physical, and social consequences for the person.

NCDs, the predominant killers of the 21st century, emerge mostly from our lifestyle as well as our social and physical environments. Industrial bioproducts in our environment and food can initiate a low-burning inflammation that might set the scene for future NCDs. Our Western diets, lifestyles, and often isolating societies (despite technological advances) seem to conspire to take us away from our need to have strong social bonds, eat healthy whole food, engage in purposeful daily activity (work and exercise), get adequate sleep, and curtail expected stressful events.

The good news is that, despite these threats to our health, emerging evidence from positive health science approaches continues to provide us with support and education that can empower us all on the journey to better health. Combining lifestyle medicine approaches with positive psychology interventions can have a synergistically positive impact on health and wellbeing. Individuals can combine traditional lifestyle medicine-based practices (sleep hygiene, eating whole food, engaging in daily physical activity, limiting alcohol consumption and avoiding tobacco smoking, and cultivating positive relationships) with positive psychology interventions (cultivating gratitude, enhancing awareness through journaling, savouring our experiences such as cooking healthy food, cultivating optimistic perspectives and a growth mindset, as well encouraging a present moment awareness through meditation and experiencing nature) for better health and wellbeing. Personalised approaches to health and wellbeing are more valued in the 21st century. There is no one-size-fits-all approach to health and wellbeing. Positive health offers individuals an extensive and ever-growing evidence-based tool kit that can be used to promote human flourishing.

However, it is imperative that the onus is not just in the individual citizen to cultivate a positive health outlook and practice for greater wellbeing. Governments (local, regional, and national), health insurers, non-governmental organisations, employers and large corporations, as well as healthcare services and systems must adopt similar strategies that are imbedded in positive health principles and practices. We must also investigate how cultural and geographical differences can influence the application of impactful positive health interventions across the world.

Our most vulnerable populations (elderly citizens living alone, lone parents, migrants, those stigmatised in our communities, the unemployed, as well as citizens isolated as a result of mental and physical disease or disabilities) must also have access to positive health tool kits that incorporate the best of positive psychology and lifestyle medicine.

## REFERENCES

Abad, V. C., & Guilleminault, C. (2003). Diagnosis and treatment of sleep disorders: A brief review for clinicians. *Dialogues in Clinical Neuroscience*, *5*(4), 371–388. https://doi.org/10.31887/DCNS.2003.5.4/vabad

ACLM. (2022). What is Lifestyle Medicine? www.lifestylemedicine.org/ACLM/ACLM/About/What_is_Lifestyle_Medicine_/Lifestyle_Medicine.aspx?hkey=26f3eb6b-8294-4a63-83de-35d429c3bb88

Ai, S. Z., & Dai, X. J. (2018). Causal role of rapid-eye-movement sleep on successful memory consolidation of fear extinction. *Journal of Thoracic Disease*, *10*(3), 1214–1216. https://doi.org/10.21037/jtd.2018.01.163

Antony, J. W., Schönauer, M., Staresina, B. P., & Cairney, S. A. (2019). Sleep spindles and memory reprocessing. *Trends in Neuroscience*, *42*(1), 1–3. https://doi.org/10.1016/j.tins.2018.09.012

Balban, M. Y., Neri, E., Kogon, M. M., Weed, L., Nouriani, B., Jo, B., ... Huberman, A. D. (2023). Brief structured respiration practices enhance mood and reduce physiological arousal. *Cell Reports Medicine*, *4*(1), 100895. https://doi.org/10.1016/j.xcrm.2022.100895

Ballesio, A., Zagaria, A., Salaris, A., Terrasi, M., Lombardo, C., & Ottaviani, C. (2023). Sleep and daily positive emotions – is heart rate variability a mediator? *Journal of Psychophysiology*, *37*(3), 134–142. https://doi.org/10.1027/0269-8803/a000315

Berisha, A., Shutkind, K., & Borniger, J. C. (2022). Sleep disruption and cancer: Chicken or the egg? *Frontiers in Neuroscience*, *16*. https://doi.org/10.3389/fnins.2022.856235

Berjaoui, C., Tesfasilassie Kibrom, B., Ghayyad, M., Joumaa, S., Talal Al Labban, N., Nazir, A., ... Uwishema, O. (2023). Unveiling the sleep–cardiovascular connection: Novel perspectives and interventions – A narrative review. *Health Science Reports*, *6*(12), e1773. https://doi.org/10.1002/hsr2.1773

Biss, R. K., & Hasher, L. (2012). Happy as a lark: Morning-type younger and older adults are higher in positive affect. *Emotion*, *12*(3), 437–441. https://doi.org/10.1037/a0027071

Blanchflower, D. G., Oswald, A. J., & Stewart-Brown, S. (2013). Is psychological well-being linked to the consumption of fruit and vegetables? *Social Indicators Research*, *114*(3), 785–801. https://doi.org/10.1007/s11205-012-0173-y

Bland, K. A., Neil-Sztramko, S. E., Zadravec, K., Medysky, M. E., Kong, J., Winters-Stone, K. M., & Campbell, K. L. (2021). Attention to principles of exercise training: An updated systematic review of randomized controlled trials in cancers other than breast and prostate. *BMC Cancer*, *21*(1), 1179. https://doi.org/10.1186/s12885-021-08701-y

Buettner, D. (2012). *The blue zones: 9 power lessons for living longer from the people who've lived the longest* (2nd ed.). National Geographic.

Buettner, D. (2024). Are supercentenarian claims based on age exaggeration? www.bluezones.com/news/are-supercentenarian-claims-based-on-age-exaggeration/

Buettner, D., & Skemp, S. (2016). Blue zones: Lessons from the world's longest lived. *American Journal of Lifestyle Medicine*, *10*(5), 318–321. https://doi.org/10.1177/1559827616637066

Burke, J., & Dunne, P. J. (2022). Lifestyle medicine pillars as predictors of psychological flourishing. *Frontiers in Psychology*, *13*, 963806. https://doi.org/10.3389/fpsyg.2022.963806

Burke, J., Dunne, P. J., Meehan, T., O'Boyle, C., & Nieuwerburgh, V. (2022). *Positive Health: 100+ research-based Positive Psychology and Lifestyle Medicine tools for enhancing wellbeing.* Routledge.

Colditz, G. A., Philpott, S. E., & Hankinson, S. E. (2016). The impact of the nurses' health study on population health: Prevention, translation, and control. *American Journal of Public Health, 106*(9), 1540–1545. https://doi.org/10.2105/ajph.2016.303343

Conner, T. S., Brookie, K. L., Richardson, A. C., & Polak, M. A. (2015). On carrots and curiosity: Eating fruit and vegetables is associated with greater flourishing in daily life. *British Journal of Health Psychology, 20*(2), 413–427. https://doi.org/10.1111/bjhp.12113

Cox, R. C., Ritchie, H. K., Knauer, O. A., Guerin, M. K., Stothard, E. R., & Wright, K. P., Jr. (2024). Chronotype and affective response to sleep restriction and subsequent sleep deprivation. *Journal of Biological Rhythms, 39*(1), 35–48. https://doi.org/10.1177/07487304231188204

Creswell, J. D. (2017). Mindfulness interventions. *Annual Review of Psychology, 68*, 491–516. https://doi.org/10.1146/annurev-psych-042716-051139

Crum, A. J., & Langer, E. J. (2007). Mind-set matters: Exercise and the placebo effect. *Psychological Science, 18*(2), 165–171. https://doi.org/10.1111/j.1467-9280.2007.01867.x

CSO (2022). Vital Statistics Yearly Summary 2022. www.cso.ie/en/releasesandpublications/ep/p-vsys/vitalstatisticsyearlysummary2022/

Czeisler, C. A., & Gooley, J. J. (2007). Sleep and circadian rhythms in humans. *Cold Spring Harbor Symposia on Quantitative Biology, 72*, 579–597. https://doi.org/10.1101/sqb.2007.72.064

Davis, A. J., MacCarron, P., & Cohen, E. (2021). Social reward and support effects on exercise experiences and performance: Evidence from parkrun. *PLOS ONE, 16*(9), e0256546. https://doi.org/10.1371/journal.pone.0256546

Divine, M. (2016). The breathing technique a Navy SEAL uses to stay calm and focused. https://time.com/4316151/breathing-technique-navy-seal-calm-focused/

Drago, V., Foster, P. S., Heilman, K. M., Aricò, D., Williamson, J., Montagna, P., & Ferri, R. (2011). Cyclic alternating pattern in sleep and its relationship to creativity. *Sleep Medicine, 12*(4), 361–366. https://doi.org/10.1016/j.sleep.2010.11.009

Drinkaware (2024). Tools and resources. www.drinkaware.ie/tools-resources/

Dunne, P. J., Lynch, J., Prihodova, L., O'Leary, C., Ghoreyshi, A., Basdeo, S. A., … Carroll, Á. (2019). Burnout in the emergency department: Randomized controlled trial of an attention-based training programmes. *Journal of Integrative Medicine, 17*(3), 173–180. https://doi.org/10.1016/j.joim.2019.03.009

Dweck, C. S., & Yeager, D. S. (2019). Mindsets: A view from two eras. *Perspectives on Psychological Science*, *14*(3), 481–496. https://doi.org/10.1177/1745691618804166

Dymock, A. (2024, 03/02/2024). What's behind teams breathing in huddle? www.rugbyworld.com/countries/australia-countries/whats-behind-the-france-and-wallabies-team-breathing-exercises-128679

Edwards, M. K., & Loprinzi, P. D. (2018). Comparative effects of meditation and exercise on physical and psychosocial health outcomes: A review of randomized controlled trials. *Postgraduate Medicine*, *130*(2), 222–228. https://doi.org/10.1080/00325481.2018.1409049

Farley, J. B., Stein, J., Keogh, J. W. L., Woods, C. T., & Milne, N. (2020). The relationship between physical fitness qualities and sport-specific technical skills in female, team-based ball players: A systematic review. *Sports Medicine Open*, *6*(1), 18. https://doi.org/10.1186/s40798-020-00245-y

Fincham, G. W., Strauss, C., Montero-Marin, J., & Cavanagh, K. (2023). Effect of breathwork on stress and mental health: A meta-analysis of randomised-controlled trials. *Scientific Reports*, *13*(1), 432. https://doi.org/10.1038/s41598-022-27247-y

Fredrickson, B. L., Cohn, M. A., Coffey, K. A., Pek, J., & Finkel, S. M. (2008). Open hearts build lives: Positive emotions, induced through loving-kindness meditation, build consequential personal resources. *Journal of Personality and Social Psychology*, *95*(5), 1045–1062. https://doi.org/10.1037/a0013262

Fritz, M. M., Armenta, C. N., Walsh, L. C., & Lyubomirsky, S. (2019). Gratitude facilitates healthy eating behavior in adolescents and young adults. *Journal of Experimental Social Psychology*, *81*, 4–14. https://doi.org/10.1016/j.jesp.2018.08.011

Garrett, N., & Sharot, T. (2017). Optimistic update bias holds firm: Three tests of robustness following Shah et al. *Consciousness and Cognition*, *50*, 12–22.

Gawrylewski, A. (2018). Be a better you (smart, happy, relaxed). *Scientific American Mind*, *27*(1), 1–112.

Glanz, K., Metcalfe, J. J., Folta, S. C., Brown, A., & Fiese, B. (2021). Diet and health benefits associated with in-home eating and sharing meals at home: A systematic review. *International Journal of Environmental Research and Public Health*, *18*(4). https://doi.org/10.3390/ijerph18041577

Gobinath, V., & Jothimani, T. (2020). Relationship between Chronotype and Happiness among Healthy Young Adults. *Indian Journal of Positive Psychology*, *11*(2), 88–92.

Gonot-Schoupinsky, F. N., Garip, G., Sheffield, D., Omar, O. M., & Arora, T. (2020). Prescribing laughter to ameliorate mental health, sleep, and wellbeing in university students: A protocol for a feasibility study of a randomised controlled trial. *Contemporary Clinical Trials Communications*, *20*, 100676. https://doi.org/10.1016/j.conctc.2020.100676

Government-of-Canada. (2024). The healthy plate as part of the healthy food guide. https://food-guide.canada.ca/en/

Hamilton, N. A., Gallagher, M. W., Preacher, K. J., Stevens, N., Nelson, C. A., Karlson, C., & McCurdy, D. (2007). Insomnia and well-being. *Journal of Consulting and Clinical Psychology*, *75*(6), 939–946.

Health Canada (2024). Canada's dietary guidelines. https://food-guide.canada.ca/en/guidelines/

Hirshkowitz, M., Whiton, K., Albert, S. M., Alessi, C., Bruni, O., DonCarlos, L., ... Ware, J. C. (2015). National Sleep Foundation's updated sleep duration recommendations: Final report. *Sleep Health*, *1*(4), 233–243. https://doi.org/10.1016/j.sleh.2015.10.004

Hitchcott, P. K., Fastame, M. C., & Penna, M. P. (2018). More to blue zones than long life: Positive psychological characteristics. *Health, Risk & Society*, *20*(3–4), 163–181. https://doi.org/10.1080/13698575.2018.1496233

Hoeppner, B. B., Hoeppner, S. S., Kelly, L., Schick, M., & Kelly, J. F. (2017). Smiling Instead of smoking: Development of a positive psychology smoking cessation smartphone app for non-daily smokers. *International Journal of Behavioral Medicine*, *24*(5), 683–693. https://doi.org/10.1007/s12529-017-9640-9

Hoeppner, B. B., Siegel, K. R., Carlon, H. A., Kahler, C. W., Park, E. R., & Hoeppner, S. S. (2021). A smoking cessation app for nondaily smokers (version 2 of the Smiling Instead of Smoking app): Acceptability and feasibility study. *JMIR Formative Research*, *5*(11), e29760. https://doi.org/10.2196/29760

HSE (2024). Quit Smoking. www2.hse.ie/living-well/quit-smoking/

Iranpour, A., & Nakhaee, N. (2019). A review of alcohol-related harms: A recent update. *Addict Health*, *11*(2), 129–137. https://doi.org/10.22122/ahj.v11i2.225

Irish, L. A., Kline, C. E., Gunn, H. E., Buysse, D. J., & Hall, M. H. (2015). The role of sleep hygiene in promoting public health: A review of empirical evidence. *Sleep Medicine Review*, *22*, 23–36. https://doi.org/10.1016/j.smrv.2014.10.001

Isaacowitz, D. M., & Seligman, M. E. (2002). Cognitive style predictors of affect change in older adults. *International Journal of Aging and Human Development*, *54*(3), 233–253. https://doi.org/10.2190/j6e5-np5k-2uc4-2f8b

Kaliman, P. (2019). Epigenetics and meditation. *Current Opinion in Psychology*, *28*, 76–80. https://doi.org/10.1016/j.copsyc.2018.11.010

Kaliman, P., Alvarez-Lopez, M. J., Cosin-Tomas, M., Rosenkranz, M. A., Lutz, A., & Davidson, R. J. (2014). Rapid changes in histone deacetylases and inflammatory gene expression in expert meditators. *Psychoneuroendocrinology*, *40*, 96–107. https://doi.org/10.1016/j.psyneuen.2013.11.004

Key, T. J., Papier, K., & Tong, T. Y. N. (2022). Plant-based diets and long-term health: Findings from the EPIC-Oxford study. *Proceedings of the Nutrition Societyy*, *81*(2), 190–198. https://doi.org/10.1017/s0029665121003748

Khan, Z., & Zadeh, Z. F. (2014). Mindful eating and it's relationship with mental well-being. *Procedia - Social and Behavioral Sciences*, *159*, 69–73. https://doi.org/10.1016/j.sbspro.2014.12.330

Killingsworth, M. A., & Gilbert, D. T. (2010). A wandering mind is an unhappy mind. *Science*, *330*(6006), 932–932. https://doi.org/10.1126/science.1192439

Kreouzi, M., Theodorakis, N., & Constantinou, C. (2022). Lessons learned from blue zones, lifestyle medicine pillars and beyond: An update on the contributions of behavior and genetics to wellbeing and longevity. *American Journal of Lifestyle Medicine*, 15598276221118494. https://doi.org/10.1177/15598276221118494

Lally, P., van Jaarsveld, C. H. M., Potts, H. W. W., & Wardle, J. (2010). How are habits formed: Modelling habit formation in the real world. *European Journal of Social Psychology*, *40*(6), 998–1009. https://doi.org/10.1002/ejsp.674

Lane, M. M., Gamage, E., Du, S., Ashtree, D. N., McGuinness, A. J., Gauci, S., ... Marx, W. (2024). Ultra-processed food exposure and adverse health outcomes: Umbrella review of epidemiological meta-analyses. *British Medical Journal*, *384*, e077310. https://doi.org/10.1136/bmj-2023-077310

Le Foll, B., Piper, M. E., Fowler, C. D., Tonstad, S., Bierut, L., Lu, L., ... Hall, W. D. (2022). Tobacco and nicotine use. *Nature Reviews Disease Primers*, *8*(1), 19. https://doi.org/10.1038/s41572-022-00346-w

Leite, F. H. M., Khandpur, N., Andrade, G. C., Anastasiou, K., Baker, P., Lawrence, M., & Monteiro, C. A. (2022). Ultra-processed foods should be central to global food systems dialogue and action on biodiversity. *BMJ Global Health*, *7*(3). https://doi.org/10.1136/bmjgh-2021-008269

Lenneis, A., Das-Friebel, A., Tang, N. K. Y., Sanborn, A. N., Lemola, S., Singmann, H., ... Realo, A. (2024). The influence of sleep on subjective wellbeing: An experience sampling study. *Emotion*, *24*(2), 451–464. https://doi.org/10.1037/emo0001268

Lianov, L. S., & Burke, J. (2025). *Lifestyle medicine from the inside out: Using positive psychology in healthy lifestyles for positive health*: Routledge.

Littman-Ovadia, H., Dubreuil, P., Meyers, M. C., & Freidlin, P. (2021). Editorial: VIA character strengths: Theory, research and practice. *Frontiers in Psychology*, *12*, 653941. https://doi.org/10.3389/fpsyg.2021.653941

Liu, Z., Guan, R., & Pan, L. (2022). Exploration of restless legs syndrome under the new concept: A review. *Medicine (Baltimore)*, *101*(50), e32324. https://doi.org/10.1097/md.0000000000032324

Loma Linda University (2024). Lifestyle Assessment Long Form. chrome-extension://efaidnbmnnnibpcajpcglclefindmkaj/https://ihacares.com/assets/pdfs/Lifestyle%20Medicine/ACLM%20LLU%20Long%20Form.pdf

Marques, P., Piqueras, L., & Sanz, M.-J. (2021). An updated overview of e-cigarette impact on human health. *Respiratory Research*, *22*(1), 151. https://doi.org/10.1186/s12931-021-01737-5

Maslach, C., & Jackson, S. E. (1981). The measurement of experienced burnout. *Journal of Organizational Behavior, 2*(2), 99–113. https://doi.org/10.1002/job.4030020205

McCambridge, J., Witton, J., & Elbourne, D. R. (2014). Systematic review of the Hawthorne effect: New concepts are needed to study research participation effects. *Journal of Clinical Epidemiology, 67*(3), 267–277. https://doi.org/10.1016/j.jclinepi.2013.08.015

McKeown, P. (2021). *The breathing cure: Exercises to develop new breathing habits for a healthier, happier and longer life.* OxyAtBooks.

McKinsey. (2022). Adding years to life and life to years. www.mckinsey.com/mhi/our-insights/adding-years-to-life-and-life-to-years

Misiąg, W., Piszczyk, A., Szymańska-Chabowska, A., & Chabowski, M. (2022). Physical activity and cancer care: A review. *Multidisciplinary Digital Publishing Institute, 14*(17), 4154. www.mdpi.com/2072-6694/14/17/4154

Moreno-Agostino, D., Caballero, F. F., Martín-María, N., Tyrovolas, S., López-García, P., Rodríguez-Artalejo, F., Haro, J. M., Ayuso-Mateos, J. L., & Miret, M. (2019). Mediterranean diet and wellbeing: Evidence from a nationwide survey. *Psychological Health, 34*(3), 321–335. https://doi.org/10.1080/08870446.2018. Epub 2018 October 15. PMID: 30320519.

Mujcic, R., & Oswald, A. J. (2016). Evolution of well-being and happiness after increases in consumption of fruit and vegetables. *American Journal of Public Health, 106*(8), 1504–1510. https://doi.org/10.2105/ajph.2016.303260

Nagata, K., Tsunoda, K., Fujii, Y., Jindo, T., & Okura, T. (2023). Impact of exercising alone and exercising with others on the risk of cognitive impairment among older Japanese adults. *Archives of Gerontology and Geriatrics, 107*, 104908. https://doi.org/10.1016/j.archger.2022.104908

Nakao, M., Shirotsuki, K., & Sugaya, N. (2021). Cognitive-behavioral therapy for management of mental health and stress-related disorders: Recent advances in techniques and technologies. *Biopsychosocial Medicine, 15*(1), 16. https://doi.org/10.1186/s13030-021-00219-w

Newman, S. J. (2024). Supercentenarian and remarkable age records exhibit patterns indicative of clerical errors and pension fraud. *bioRxiv*, 704080. https://doi.org/10.1101/704080

Orlich, M. J., Singh, P. N., Sabaté, J., Jaceldo-Siegl, K., Fan, J., Knutsen, S., … Fraser, G. E. (2013). Vegetarian dietary patterns and mortality in Adventist Health Study 2. *JAMA Internal Medicine, 173*(13), 1230–1238. https://doi.org/10.1001/jamainternmed.2013.6473

Palmer, C. A., Bower, J. L., Cho, K. W., Clementi, M. A., Lau, S., Oosterhoff, B., & Alfano, C. A. (2024). Sleep loss and emotion: A systematic review and meta-analysis of over 50 years of experimental research. *Psychological Bulletin, 150*(4), 440–463. https://doi.org/10.1037/bul0000410

Patel, A. K. R. V.; Shumway, K.R.; Araujo, J.F. (2024). Physiology, sleep stages. www.ncbi.nlm.nih.gov/books/NBK526132/

Patke, A., Young, M. W., & Axelrod, S. (2020). Molecular mechanisms and physiological importance of circadian rhythms. *Nature Reviews Molecular Cell Biology*, *21*(2), 67–84. https://doi.org/10.1038/s41580-019-0179-2

Peever, J., & Fuller, P. M. (2016). Neuroscience: A distributed neural network controls REM Sleep. *Current Biology*, *26*(1), R34–35. https://doi.org/10.1016/j.cub.2015.11.011

Pes, G. M., Dore, M. P., Tsofliou, F., & Poulain, M. (2022). Diet and longevity in the blue zones: A set-and-forget issue? *Maturitas*, *164*, 31–37. https://doi.org/10.1016/j.maturitas.2022.06.004

Phelan, C. H., Love, G. D., Ryff, C. D., Brown, R. L., & Heidrich, S. M. (2010). Psychosocial predictors of changing sleep patterns in aging women: A multiple pathway approach. *Psychological Aging*, *25*(4), 858–866. https://doi.org/10.1037/a0019622

Piercy, K. L., Troiano, R. P., Ballard, R. M., Carlson, S. A., Fulton, J. E., Galuska, D. A., ... Olson, R. D. (2018). The physical activity guidelines for Americans. *JAMA*, *320*(19), 2020–2028. https://doi.org/10.1001/jama.2018.14854

Pollan, M. (2009). *In defense of food: An eater's manifesto* (1st ed.). Penguin Books.

Positive Psychology Center (2024). Questionnaires for researchers. https://ppc.sas.upenn.edu/resources/questionnaires-researchers

Poulain, M., Herm, A., & Pes, G. (2013). The blue zones: Areas of exceptional longevity around the world. *Vienna Yearbook of Population Research*, *11*, 87–108.

Punjabi, N. M. (2008). The epidemiology of adult obstructive sleep apnea. *Proceedings of the American Thoracic Society*, *5*(2), 136–143. https://doi.org/10.1513/pats.200709-155MG

Ridge, K., Conlon, N., Hennessy, M., & Dunne, P. J. (2021). Feasibility assessment of an 8-week attention-based training programme in the management of chronic spontaneous urticaria. *Pilot and Feasibility Studies*, 7(1), 103. https://doi.org/10.1186/s40814-021-00841-z

Roepke, A. M., Jayawickreme, E., & Riffle, O. M. (2014). Meaning and health: A systematic review. *Applied Research in Quality of Life*, *9*(4), 10551079. https://doi.org/10.1007/s11482-013-9288-9

Ryff, C. D., Singer, B. H., & Dienberg Love, G. (2004). Positive health: Connecting wellbeing with biology. *Philosophical Transactions of the Royal Society London B: Biological Sciences*, *359*(1449), 1383–1394. https://doi.org/10.1098/rstb.2004.1521

Sandhu, A., Seth, M., & Gurm, H. S. (2014). Daylight savings time and myocardial infarction. *Open Heart*, *1*(1), e000019. https://doi.org/10.1136/openhrt-2013-000019

Sapolsky, R. M. (2004). *Why zebras don't get ulcers*. New York: Times Books.

Schulz, H., Bes, E., & Jobert, M. (1997). Modelling sleep propensity and sleep disturbances. In K. Meier-Ewert & M. Okawa (Eds.), *Sleep–Wake Disorders* (pp. 11–26). Springer US.

Schulz, P., & Steimer, T. (2009). Neurobiology of circadian systems. *CNS Drugs, 23 Suppl 2*, 3–13. https://doi.org/10.2165/11318620-000000000-00000

Scott, A. J., Webb, T. L., Martyn-St James, M., Rowse, G., & Weich, S. (2021). Improving sleep quality leads to better mental health: A meta-analysis of randomised controlled trials. *Sleep Medicine Review, 60*, 101556. https://doi.org/10.1016/j.smrv.2021.101556

Singer, T., & Engert, V. (2019). It matters what you practice: Differential training effects on subjective experience, behavior, brain and body in the ReSource Project. *Current Opinion in Psychology, 28*, 151–158. https://doi.org/10.1016/j.copsyc.2018.12.005

Stanisławska Kubiak, M., Wójciak, R. W., Trzeszczyńska, N., Czajeczny, D., Samborski, W., & Mojs, E. (2019). Who is happier: Smoker or non-smoker? Smoking in medical students from the perspective of positive psychology. *Eurpean Review of Medicine Pharmacological Science, 23*(5), 2174–2181. https://doi.org/10.26355/eurrev_201903_17263

Steger, M. F. (2017). Meaning in life and wellbeing. In M. Slade, L. Oades, & A. Jarden (Eds.), *Wellbeing, Recovery and Mental Health* (pp. 75–85). Cambridge: Cambridge University Press.

Steptoe, A., Dockray, S., & Wardle, J. (2009). Positive affect and psychobiological processes relevant to health. *Journal of Personality, 77*(6), 1747–1776. https://doi.org/10.1111/j.1467-6494.2009.00599.x

Tan, M. N., Mevsim, V., Pozlu Cifci, M., Sayan, H., Ercan, A. E., Ergin, O. F., … Ensari, S. (2020). Who is happier among preclinical medical students: The impact of chronotype preference. *Chronobiology International, 37*(8), 1163–1172. https://doi.org/10.1080/07420528.2020.1761373

Uchino, B. N., Cribbet, M., de Grey, R. G., Cronan, S., Trettevik, R., & Smith, T. W. (2017). Dispositional optimism and sleep quality: A test of mediating pathways. *Journal of Behavioral Medicine, 40*(2), 360–365. https://doi.org/10.1007/s10865-016-9792-0

US Department of Veterans Affairs, V. (2022). Recharging through the Personal Health Inventory. www.va.gov/WHOLEHEALTH/features/Recharging_With_PHI.asp

Veronese, N., Solmi, M., Caruso, M. G., Giannelli, G., Osella, A. R., Evangelou, E., … Tzoulaki, I. (2018). Dietary fiber and health outcomes: An umbrella review of systematic reviews and meta-analyses. *American Journal of Clinical Nutrition, 107*(3), 436–444. https://doi.org/10.1093/ajcn/nqx082

Walker, J., Muench, A., Perlis, M. L., & Vargas, I. (2022). Cognitive behavioral therapy for insomnia (CBT-I): A Primer. *Kliničeskaâ i special'naâ psihologiâ*, *11*(2), 123–137. https://doi.org/10.17759/cpse.2022110208

Warner, R., Frye, K., Morrell, J., & Carey, G. (2017). Fruit and vegetable intake predicts positive affect. *Journal of Happiness Studies*, *18*. https://doi.org/10.1007/s10902-016-9749-6

Weitzer, J., Papantoniou, K., Lázaro-Sebastià, C., Seidel, S., Klösch, G., & Schernhammer, E. (2021). The contribution of dispositional optimism to understanding insomnia symptomatology: Findings from a cross-sectional population study in Austria. *Journal of Sleep Research*, *30*(1), e13132. https://doi.org/10.1111/jsr.13132

West, R. (2017). Tobacco smoking: Health impact, prevalence, correlates and interventions. *Psychology & Health*, *32*(8), 1018–1036. https://doi.org/10.1080/08870446.2017.1325890

WHO. (2020). *WHO guidelines on physical activity and sedentary behaviour*. http://www.ncbi.nlm.nih.gov/books/NBK566045/

WHO. (2022). Physical activity (Key Facts). www.who.int/news-room/fact-sheets/detail/physical-activity

Yasuma, F., & Hayano, J. (2004). Respiratory sinus arrhythmia: Why does the heartbeat synchronize with respiratory rhythm? *Chest*, *125*(2), 683–690. https://doi.org/10.1378/chest.125.2.683

Yordanova, J., Kolev, V., Wagner, U., & Verleger, R. (2010). Differential associations of early- and late-night sleep with functional brain states promoting insight to abstract task regularity. *PLOS ONE*, *5*(2), e9442. https://doi.org/10.1371/journal.pone.0009442

# POSITIVE ENVIRONMENT AND HEALTH

There are diverse ways in which health and wellbeing are understood and studied across different disciplines, particularly psychology and economics. These are important to understand as different perspectives shape our understanding of wellbeing and influence public policies, priorities, and services. As stated earlier in this book, positive health perceives health as a state of wellbeing rather than a state of illness and incorporates a shift towards perceiving body and mind as an integrated system (O'Boyle et al., 2024). This chapter explores further how we can conceptualise "an integrated system".

Well-being can be viewed differently across disciplines and over time. Traditionally, within the Western psychology perspective, wellbeing was measured by the absence of illness, resulting in an unbalanced view of human beings – sick versus not sick. Positive psychology emerged as a movement to shift the focus towards what is right with people (Seligman & Csikszentmihalyi, 2000) and to explore the positive aspects of wellbeing, not just deficits (Burke & Arslan, 2020), and what makes life worth living (Peterson et al., 2008). In positive psychology, the overall state of flourishing and fulfilment in an individual's life matters – with positive emotions, engagement, relationships, meaning and purpose, and accomplishment being examples of elements needed to thrive and flourish. In lifestyle medicine (Sagner et al., 2017) wellbeing is viewed as the overall health and quality of life achieved through a balance of various lifestyle factors, including healthy eating, physical activity, stress management, sleep, avoiding alcohol and tobacco, as well as cultivating positive social connections. From these

DOI: 10.4324/9781003457169-6

more recent developments wellbeing is generally now considered to encompass not just the absence of disease, but also the presence of positive physical, mental, and social outcomes, allowing individuals to thrive and reach their full potential. However, there are criticisms of these conceptualisations of wellbeing, namely that they often fail to account for cultural differences and the perspectives of marginalised individuals.

Additionally, as Bilbao-Nieva and Meyer (2024) note, wellbeing conceptualisation should not be seen as apolitical. They illustrate this by giving examples of ethical consequences of assessing happiness and wellbeing as self-reported views that reproduce certain social behaviours or expectations that are believed to cause happiness, for example marriage (quoting Ahmed, 2010), but which may not and may even reproduce social systems that are not necessarily progressive. They also quote Cabanas and Illouz (2019) who question positive psychology's approach to wellbeing as something an individual can achieve themselves without recognising the importance of living conditions and social justice. Cultural factors, such as individual or collective agency and spirituality (Carreno et al., 2023; Chirico, 2016; Wong, 2011) significantly impact wellbeing. Additionally, marginalised individuals may have different conceptualisations of wellbeing compared to those in mainstream society and are not often included in wellbeing measures (Muthukrishna et al., 2020). A greater focus on living conditions and human rights would also be argued from a developmental economics approach. We will return to these criticisms later in the chapter, but within all these conceptualisations the environment can inhibit, promote, or in some way influence wellbeing.

We have already seen from Chapter 4 that we as individuals are in constant contact with our physical environment and that "our physical health is dependent on how polluted or clean our environment is, the temperature of the climate, the nature of the food we eat and purity of the air we breathe" (Burket et al., 2024). In this chapter we illustrate how the interaction or interfacing of people with the environment in lifestyle medicine and positive psychology influences people's wellbeing. These examples are based on the built, natural, social, and cultural environment, but other examples, such as the work, technological, and political environments could equally have been used. We then go beyond these examples to suggest a more interconnected and interdependent view of well-being and the environment that we propose fits better with our understanding of positive health. This is a view of the mutual reliance and entwining of different components of the environment, where humans have and play an essential role in maintaining the integrity and functionality of the whole but are "intra-connected" with the world we live in. This is explored through the idea of relational approaches to wellbeing, which focus on the interconnectedness between individuals, their environments, and social structures and help us understand the contextuality of wellbeing.

## WELL-BEING AND THE ENVIRONMENT WITHIN LIFESTYLE MEDICINE AND POSITIVE PSYCHOLOGY

In lifestyle medicine, the environment is considered broadly as the external factors and conditions that influence lifestyle behaviours; for example, the physical environment (such as the natural and built environments) and the social environment (such as support networks and socioeconomic conditions). Lifestyle medicine advocates for creating supportive environments that promote healthy behaviours and prevent chronic diseases as the environmental factors interact with individual lifestyle choices and behaviours to impact health outcomes. Creating these environments may involve interventions at various levels and across sectors, such as policy changes for improved infrastructure, better choice of food in supermarkets in socio-economically disadvantaged areas and better primary school education on healthy lifestyles. In a similar way, positive psychology considers environment as the external context or surroundings that influence a person's wellbeing. This includes physical surroundings, social interactions, cultural norms, and broader societal factors. However, rather than focusing on preventing poor health outcomes in terms of promoting positive lifestyle choices, positive psychology emphasises the crucial role that the environment plays in shaping a person's physical, psychological, and physiological wellbeing. For example, negative environments can cause or create stress or limit growth, whereas supportive environments can provide resources and opportunities to thrive and flourish. In relation to the emphasis on positive emotions in positive psychology, Ryff (2022) has expressed concern this can lead to a superficial and overly simplistic understanding of wellbeing.

She has argued that wellbeing is a complex and dynamic construct that involves both positive and negative emotions, as well as a sense of meaning and purpose in life. Wellbeing isn't just about feeling happy; it's about the whole experience, including pain and discomfort. Wellbeing arises from everything around us – objects, smells, language, structures, beliefs – both positive and negative.

A supportive "built environment" can encourage physical activity, outdoor recreation, and healthy behaviours, while an unhealthy environment may discourage or hinder such activities. According to Prof Donal O' Shea (Earth Horizon, 2018) we are living in an obesogenic world where it is hard to make the right lifestyle choices, given how the roads are built, the lighting that is provided, the availability of public transport, and the types of food that are affordable and accessible. Environmental design of cities, such as the availability of safe footpaths and ease of access to shops and services, can be a major contributor to people walking and exercising more (Sallis et al., 2016), whereas in rural or peri-urban areas poorly lit footpaths and few services close to home act as barriers to exercise (Ferguson et al., 2016). Urban residents may encounter social isolation as a consequence of heightened urban density and heterogeneity within their neighbourhoods, coupled with inadequate public spaces for residents to gather, interact and form relationships (Baur et al., 2013). In many cases the same built environment can be viewed and experienced differently, and hence divergently impact multiple dimensions of individuals wellbeing. For example, women may not be, or not feel, safe walking streets whereas men living in the same area may be or may feel very safe. In a study by Adelson in India (Adelson et al., 2016, 2017) women feared being grabbed, sexually assaulted, or threatened on the streets. This did not just have an impact on physical activity, but also on family relationships, especially when the women were blamed or held responsible for those actions by family members.

Environments perceived as safe and secure foster a sense of physical and psychological wellbeing, enabling individuals to engage in activities with confidence and freedom from fear. The absence of perceived threats or hazards within the environment enables a more relaxed state and facilitates the restoration of cognitive resources, thereby enhancing individuals' overall quality of life. The importance of planning and designing and how it affects people's health, especially in low and middle-income countries, is emphasised by Smit and colleagues (Smit et al., 2011). Urban planning and design influence things like access to housing, infrastructure, and healthy environments, which can impact people's health and wellbeing and health equity (Smit et al., 2011). Positive psychology underscores the importance of access to restorative environments in promoting psychological resilience and mitigating the detrimental effects of chronic stress.

### Forest-bathing/Shinrin Yoku

*Mayumi had moved to England with her daughter a few years ago from Japan. She often took care of her grandson when her daughter went out to work. She took her role as custodian and teacher of her grandson in their culture and practice seriously. Mayumi was also very practiced in the ways of passing on intergenerational knowledge.*

*One morning she gently clasped her grandson Kenji's hand as they walked through the dense forest on a bright autumn day. The air was crisp, filled with the scent of pine and damp leaves. Kenji's shoulders were slumped, his brows furrowed in frustration. He had been engrossed in an online game with his friends when Mayumi insisted they go for a walk.*

*"O-ba-chan (Granny), why do we have to do this?" Kenji grumbled, kicking a pebble off the path.*

*Mayumi smiled, her eyes crinkling at the corners. "Kenji, this is a special practice called shinrin yoku, or forest bathing. It's a way to relax and connect with nature." Kenji sighed, looking unconvinced. "But I was in the middle of a game with my friends." Mayumi stopped walking and turned to face him. "I understand, Kenji. But being in nature is important for our health and wellbeing. It helps us de-stress and feel more peaceful. Let me show you how."*

*Reluctantly, Kenji nodded. Mayumi led him deeper into the forest, the sound of their footsteps softened by the carpet of fallen leaves. "First", she said, "turn off your phone. This will help you relax and be aware of your surroundings." Kenji pulled out his phone and turned it off, slipping it into his pocket. "Okay", he stated.*

*"Slow down", Mayumi instructed. "Move through the forest slowly so you can see and feel more." Kenji followed her lead, matching her slow pace. They walked in silence for a few moments, and Mayumi continued, "Take long breaths deep down into your stomach. Breathe*

in through your nose, and then slowly exhale. Make the breathing out twice as long as your breathing in." Kenji giggled at first, looking at his granny walking along calmly breathing in and out, in and out. He then mimicked his grandmother's deep breathing, feeling the cool air fill his lungs and began to feel a sense of calm arising inside him.

"Stop here for a moment", Mayumi said, coming to a halt beside a moss-covered rock. "Stand still, close your eyes, and smell what's around you. What can you smell?" Kenji closed his eyes and took a deep breath. "I smell pine and the soil", he said. "Good", Mayumi replied. "Now, open your eyes wide, use all of your senses – see, listen, smell, taste and touch." Kenji opened his eyes wide and looked around. He saw the sunlight filtering through the trees, creating dappled patterns on the forest floor. He heard the distant call of a bird and the rustling of leaves in the breeze. She waited a few moments and asked, "How do you feel?" "It feels peaceful", he admitted, "I feel peaceful".

"Before we go back let's sit quietly for a while", Mayumi suggested, guiding him to a fallen log. "Try to just think about where we are now and our surroundings, not the plans you have later with your friends or what you are going to eat for dinner". They sat together in silence, listening to the noises of the forest. Kenji spotted a squirrel scampering up a tree and a butterfly fluttering nearby. " O-ba-chan, this is actually nice", he said softly. Mayumi smiled warmly.

As they continued their walk, Kenji felt an appreciation for the peace he had found in the forest. He realised that, while he loved playing games with his friends, there was something nice about being in nature with his grandmother. It was a different kind of connection, more calming and peaceful that he had been for some time. By the time they returned home, Kenji felt lighter, his mind clearer. He looked at Mayumi with gratitude. "Thank you, Grandma. I think I needed this." Mayumi hugged him gently. "Remember, Kenji, nature is always here for you. Whenever you need to relax and find peace, just come back to the forest." Kenji nodded, feeling a bond with his grandmother and the forest that he knew he would cherish forever.

Adapted from: Forestry England, Your Guide to Forest bathing (www.forestryengland.uk/blog/forest-bathing#:~:text=What%20is%20forest%20bathing%3F,wellbeing%20in%20a%20natural%20way)

Growing evidence to suggest that being in nature – "the natural environment" – has positive effects on people's mental health. Walking in nature can have significant cognitive gains, as well as improving moods (Berman et al., 2012). Studies have shown that green spaces can lower levels of stress (Wells & Evans, 2003) and reduce rates of depression and anxiety, reduce cortisol levels (Park et al., 2010) and improve general wellbeing. Green spaces can provide a buffer against the negative health impacts of stressful life events. A Dutch study showed that residents with a higher area of green spaces within a 3 km radius had a better relationship with stressful life events (van den Berg et al., 2010). Simply being in nature or forest bathing (*Shinrin-yoku*) can improve wellbeing (Ideno et al., 2017; Park et al., 2010; Wen et al., 2019). A study involving 20,000 participants, conducted by Mathew White and his team at the European Centre for Environment & Human Health, University of Exeter (White et al., 2013), found that individuals living in urban areas with more green space tend to report greater wellbeing than city dwellers that don't have parks, gardens, or other green space nearby. Perhaps more remarkably is that the beneficial influence of green space exposure on the development of behavioural problems and cognitive function has been indicated in children as young as four years of age (Dockx et al., 2022). Reflecting on the evolution of this topic, Richard Louv, a journalist based in San Diego and author of *Last Child in the Woods* (Louv, 2008) noted the significance of his work in igniting discussions around what is often described as "Nature Deficit Disorder".

---

### THREE GOOD THINGS IN NATURE

#### (Adapted from Keenan et al., 2021)

If you live in a rural area, walk to a forest, park, beach, mountain, lakeside, or bog area for half an hour every day for five consecutive days. If you live in an urban area, walk through a housing estate, town centre, town park, or along a main road. Try to vary your walk each day. You can go alone, with another person, or with a group. As you walk daily, try to notice three good things in nature. Then, when you are in the company of others, share the three things you noticed. Apart from improving wellbeing and encouraging people to do physical activity, this tool is associated with reduced anxiety and depression.

Positive psychology acknowledges that the aesthetic appeal of the physical environment has the capacity to induce relaxation and influence individuals' psychological states and overall satisfaction with life. Aesthetics play a fundamental role in shaping individuals' perceptions and emotional responses to their surroundings (Mastandrea et al., 2019). Environments characterised by visually pleasing elements, such as natural landscapes or well-designed urban spaces, give rise to feelings of tranquillity, pleasure, and connectedness to nature (Leddy, 2015; Løvoll et al., 2020). As such, nature influences brain function, stress reduction, immune system function, mood regulation, and overall health. Selhub and Logan, in their book *Your Brain on Nature* (Selhub & Logan, 2012), give examples of how to incorporate nature into your daily life in some simple ways, such as placing plants in the office, getting a pet, and walking in nature to promote optimal health and vitality. Settings that facilitate relaxation, such as parks, gardens, or tranquil natural landscapes, offer respite from the demands of daily life and enable individuals to unwind and recharge.

---

### CONNECTING TO NATURE

**(Adapted from Passmore & Holder, 2017; Passmore et al., 2022)**

Over the next two weeks, be mindful of how the natural environment you encounter daily makes you feel. If any specific place evokes powerful emotions in you, take a photograph or make a note about it with as much detail as you can think of.

---

One increasingly debated topic around the natural environment is not just the lack of being in nature, but the loss of human connection with it – the connection being replaced or eroded by a virtual environment. This is something that Selhub and Logan (2012) also raise in reaction to the ubiquitous influence of everyday technology on the brain, and how this can potentially overload and even change the brain. Furthermore, with the increasing lack of connection with the natural environment, the value of traditional ecological knowledge and ways of living in promoting respect and awareness of environmental sustainability and wellbeing is being lost. This is having negative impacts on people's health and wellbeing. *If Women Rose*

*Rooted*, a book written by Irish author and activist, Sharon Blackie (2016), draws on mythology, folklore, and the author's own experiences in describing the historical and cultural role of the land in women's lives in Ireland and the importance of reconnecting with the natural world. Blackie argue that women's disconnection from the natural world is a key factor in the environmental and social crises facing the world today. She explores the role of myth and folklore in shaping women's relationships with the land and argues that these stories can inspire and empower women today. Women are encouraged to reconnect with the natural world through practices such as gardening, foraging, and wild swimming, and to see themselves as part of a larger ecological system. This call is not just for the benefit of women, as Blackie argues that the reclamation of women's connection to the land is a key element in the creation of a more just and sustainable society.

### Tendai Moyo

*In a small village, there lived a young woman named Tendai Moyo. Tendai was born with HIV and had lost her parents and two siblings at a young age. Now 18, she felt trapped by her circumstances, struggling to see any hope for a fulfilling life. She had left school at 14 and made a meagre living by cleaning houses in the wealthier areas nearby. Tendai's life was hard, and she often felt alone and hopeless. Tendai had been prescribed antiretroviral therapy (ART) from a young age, but she found it difficult to take her medication regularly – what was the point when she was going to die anyway? She feared that people would reject and discriminate against her if they knew she was HIV positive, so she kept her status a secret, hiding her struggles from the world.*

*In the same village, there was a friendly woman named Farai, who was a counsellor for a local NGO. Farai was the same age as Tendai and had a warm, compassionate heart. She often saw Tendai sitting alone on a bench under the tree on the outskirts of the village. One day, Farai approached Tendai and suggested she join a support group for young people living with HIV. Tendai was hesitant and afraid that joining the group would expose her secret to everyone in the village. Understanding Tendai's fears, Farai didn't push her. Instead, she began to visit Tendai regularly, sitting with her on the bench and chatting about life, their daily routines, and village activities. Tendai found these conversations surprisingly comforting. She realised that talking with Farai was easy because she didn't have to hide any part of her life. One day, Farai mentioned a new programme focusing on HIV and self-worth that was starting in a nearby town. She encouraged Tendai to enrol, assuring her that the bus fare would be covered by the organisers. After some thought, Tendai decided to give it a try.*

*Over the next few weeks, Tendai attended the programme and began to learn about herself—her beliefs, her fears, and her desires. Her confidence started to grow, and she began to forgive herself and her late mother, whom she had blamed for infecting her with HIV. For the first time, Tendai visited her mother's grave and placed flowers there, feeling a sense of peace she had never known. Tendai also asked her own body for forgiveness for not taking care of it properly. She realised that she had been neglecting her health out of fear and self-stigma. As she participated in the programmes, she discovered a love for creative activities, especially singing. She had enjoyed singing as a child but had stopped attending choir for fear of being stigmatised. Now, with renewed confidence and hope, Tendai began to think about joining a choir again. She even considered going back to school or finding a better job. Her life started to feel full of possibilities. Though she had not yet disclosed her HIV status to many members of her extended family, she felt that one day soon, she might be ready to do so.*

*Tendai's journey was just beginning, but she had already taken significant steps toward a brighter, more hopeful future. With Farai's support and the lessons she had learned about self-worth and acceptance, Tendai began to believe in herself and the life she could build. She knew there would be challenges ahead, but she also knew she had the strength to face them, and that made all the difference.*

For more information on the programme Tendai participated in see Ferris France et al. (2023) and the Beyond Stigma website (www.beyondstigma.org/wakakosha).

Social norms, cultural practices, and peer influences – the "social environment" – can either encourage, maintain, or discourage healthy lifestyle habits. One example of social norms that negatively impacts both flourishing and lifestyle habits is stigma. Stigma emerges from a dynamic social process that is enacted and perpetuated through structures, organisations, communities, and individuals (Stangl et al., 2013). Byrne et al. have conducted research with colleagues around stigma, self-stigma in particular, and we often find that, stemming from the stigma in society (the social stigma), many people internalise these negative beliefs, attitudes, and behaviours (self-stigma). Self-stigma can result in feelings of shame, worthlessness, and self-blame, and impacts social interaction, mental health, and health service utilisation. In Zimbabwe, an intervention to move young people and adolescents living with HIV from self-stigma to self-worth was designed – *Wakakosha* (you are worth it) (Ferris France et al., 2023). At its core was Inquiry-Based Stress Reduction (IBSR) (https://thework.com/) – a unique way of identifying and questioning deeply rooted self-stigma, combined with mindfulness, meditation, and creativity. The intervention had transformative effects around self-judgement, self-worth, self-agency, self-esteem, body positivity, self-forgiveness, and forgiveness of others. What was also highlighted was that culturally and practically, interventions to improve self-worth and reduce self-stigma should operate at various levels of our environment (Ferris-France et al, 2023). To address self-stigma we need to look at the connection between individual, family, community, and social levels in the environment, so understanding contemporary social pathology, the study of social issues, problems, and health conditions within our society, is particularly important in dealing with stigma. This extends beyond people living with HIV. For example, individuals experiencing homelessness or mental illness or migrancy may face stigma due to societal perceptions. Stigma can also exacerbate social pathology by creating barriers in accessing resources, support, and opportunities for affected individuals or groups, leading to social exclusion, discrimination, and marginalisation, further perpetuating the cycle of social problems.

In addition to the more tangible effects of our environment, increasing attention is being given to how our surroundings connect to our communities and who we are. The work of June Bam Hutchison explores the recapturing of our "cultural environment" that has often been shaped, recreated, or erased for particular political agendas. In her book *Ausi Told Me: Why Cape Herstoriographies Matter* (Bam, 2021), Bam explores the significance of Cape herstoriographies, narratives that challenge traditional historical accounts by placing the experiences and perspectives of marginalised groups at the centre. This is illustrated through stories, memories, and oral histories of the "Ausi", or ordinary women in Cape Town, South Africa, whose voices have been historically excluded from mainstream historical narratives. Bam recognises that people's lives are influenced by race, gender, class, sexuality, ability, and more, and that these aspects of identity cannot be examined separately, but intersect and interact in complex ways. Through this intersectional lens, Bam examines how race, class, gender, and other social factors shape the lived experiences of Cape Town's inhabitants, contribute to a subtler understanding of the city's complex history and impact the inhabitant's wellbeing and self-identity. Bam believes that these historical stories are essential for understanding and promoting social justice, reclaiming lost narratives, and fostering a more inclusive and representative historiography. These cultural norms, traditions, beliefs, and values also influence lifestyle choices related to diet, physical activity, smoking, alcohol consumption, and stress management as well as our wellbeing.

Interestingly, countries outside Europe and North Amercia have often adopted Western models of wellbeing without changing or contextualising them; e.g. Prinsloo et al. (2016) examined the wellbeing of HIV patients in Africa. However, there's a noticeable trend towards customising these models to incorporate the unique characteristics of distinct cultures, such as more collectivist societies (for example Lai, 2022; Tam et al., 2012). Some new models of flourishing tailored to reflect the diverse cultural backgrounds of populations have emerged. For instance, the Flourish Index (FI) and Secure Flourish Index (SFI) have been developed to accommodate non-Western conceptualisations of flourishing. Dambi et al. (2022) are conducting a review to conceptualise and conduct a psychometric evaluation of positive psychological outcome measures used in adolescents and young adults living with in sub-Saharan Africa. In addition to models and measures being contextualised, scholars like Guse (2022) have identified a number of positive psychology interventions in Africa, but advocates for their adaptation to different cultural practices and traditions.

Cultural factors, such as individual or collective agency and spirituality (Carreno et al., 2023; Chirico, 2016; Wong, 2011), significantly impact wellbeing. Cultural practices such as mindfulness, gratitude exercises, and acts of kindness create a positive emotional climate and vary across communities. Additionally, marginalised individuals in any culture may have different conceptualisations of wellbeing compared to those in mainstream society. Cultural differences in self-perception, as outlined in Markus and Kitayama's model of self (1991), further contribute to diverse perspectives on wellbeing. Independent selves are promoted and more active in social science research and largely include those who are Western/Global North; men; white; middle class (measured by education level); Protestant; and working in business corporate settings. Interdependent selves largely include those who are Eastern/Global South; women; black and brown people; working class (measured by education level); Catholic, Jewish; and working in non-governmental organisations. Research around wellbeing and its assessment has been privileged by the independent self. The independent concept of the self tends to totalise our identity and sense of self to the exclusion of the social, spiritual, and self-transcendent aspects of self.

Recently, a lexicography of words outside the English language relating to wellbeing was created (Lomas, 2016, 2021). The author searched for words from various cultures that describe different aspects of wellbeing, including positive feelings, ambivalent feelings, love, prosociality, character, spirituality, cognition, embodiment, aesthetics, eco-connection, competence, and understanding. The breadth and depth of these words and their meanings highlight the limited perspective that the Western conceptualisation of wellbeing offers. For example, the lexicography explores seven languages that have a word describing mixed feelings, such as Greek's *Charmolypi*, indicating a mixture of sadness and happiness; Czech's *Krasosmutněn*, implying beautiful sadness, and Dutch's *Weemoed*, indicating the strength to overcome sorrow. These examples highlight the importance of considering wellbeing from various cultural perspectives. Overall, our current definitions of wellbeing are predominantly informed by a small segment of the global population which is individual centred. A more inclusive approach that respects diverse cultural backgrounds is required in conceptualising wellbeing, developing culturally sensitive measures in assessing flourishing, and designing effective positive health interventions.

Cultural norms, traditions, beliefs, and values also impact our built environment and the designing of our services. The healthcare system is a good example of this. Most of the global north has a health system designed based on a biomedical system – a disease care rather than a health care model, though there is an increasing, but small recognition of the mind–body connection – the gut–brain axis – in the designing and delivery of services. However, as Ibeneme and colleagues (Ibeneme et al., 2017) note, ethnomedical beliefs about the causes of illness give rise to a very different understanding of wellbeing, ill health, and treatment in much of the Global South. They note that in rural areas in lower income countries, where a large proportion of the population resides, knowledge of health and illness has evolved over centuries of practice and knowledge. Traditional medicine is often the most accessible and affordable healthcare system. The two medical systems represent and are influenced by the cultural environment in which they exist, and are shaped in terms of cultural beliefs, traditional practices, and social relationships. The biomedical system is very effective in treating acute diseases, but less so for chronic diseases where there are many factors contributing to the disease and the long-term management of disease. In their discussion of how our wellbeing decisions are informed by our experiences, advice from family and friends, cultural beliefs, and professional knowledge, Ibeneme and colleagues (Ibeneme et al., 2017) postulate that no single medical system can cover all these aspects. They therefore argue that it is important for different healthcare systems to work together in cultural communities. Understanding how culture and healing intersect is crucial for improving health. Instead of keeping these systems separate, we should focus on bringing them together to overcome health challenges and existing resources strains that the biomedical model is facing in most countries.

### Recognising herbal remedies

*For generations, herbal remedies had been a tradition in our family. The knowledge of plants and their healing properties was handed down from father to son, mother to daughter – everyone in the family was involved. My mother, sisters, and I all practised it. My great-great-grandfather was particularly renowned for his treatment of osteoarthritis, and people came from far and wide to seek his remedies.*

*When my father was young, he suffered a severe injury that damaged his brain cells. The doctors in the hospital gave him a year to live and administered ether. Determined to survive, he left the hospital* and returned home, where he began treating himself with our family's herbal remedies – remedies that were part and parcel of the place. He used herbs both internally and externally to cleanse his body and heal his wounds. Remarkably, he recovered, defying all medical expectations. People saw the transformation in him and started coming to see him for help.

Nowadays, most people come to me with stress-related conditions. While I don't claim to cure diseases – if I had a cure for something like rheumatoid arthritis I'd have people from all over the world coming to see me – I offer treatments that ease pain and provide comfort. These remedies can complement modern medicine. Sometimes, though, I must tell people I can't assist them, as not every ailment can be treated with herbs.

Most of my knowledge was handed down from my father, though I did receive some formal training. Initially, I was studying agriculture, but I decided to leave my studies to learn directly from my father. It was a transformative experience. I learned not just the scientific aspects of herbalism, but also the art and intuition that come with years of practice.

Later, my father fell ill again and developed Parkinson's disease. I saw firsthand the combined benefits of modern medicine and his own herbal remedies. Despite his illness, he continued to see people every day, never complaining. Through him, I learned compassion and tolerance. I worked closely with him, and gradually, people began to trust me as much as they trusted him. That's how I started.

In this way, our family's tradition of herbal medicine continues. We recognise the value of combining conventional and traditional practices to enhance health and wellbeing. The journey of healing is ongoing, evolving with each generation, blending old wisdom with new knowledge.

Created from an interview between David Hanly and Seán Boylan on "Hanly's People", broadcast on 14 November 1988 and available at www.rte.ie/archives/2023/1101/1414104-sean-boylan-herbalist/

An applied example of linking biomedical and traditional health systems can be illustrated in the work Byrne et al. was involved with many years ago in an eastern province of South Africa when I was working with UNICEF and the uThukela District Child

Survival Project. Byrne et al. were trying to address a large number of preventable childhood illnesses by understanding cultural practices around child-rearing – building on positive practices and reframing or changing the more negative ones. Following discussions with mothers, fathers, grandmothers, traditional leaders, children and young people, and health professionals, some of the traditional beliefs and practices were relatively easy to incorporate into the standard methods promoted by the health facilities and vice versa. For example, the traditional healers were supplied and used the oral rehydration salt (ORS) packages from UNICEF to treat dehydrated children as this was often the first port of call for carers of sick children. Another was where women traditionally would express all their milk if the mother had been separated from the baby for an extended period of time, and the baby then missed out on this feed. This was changed by agreeing that only a small amount ("one tot") would need to be expressed, and in this way the mothers would still have sufficient breastmilk to feed their babies, and the practice would still be in keeping with local beliefs and practices (Byrne & Gregory, 2007). This work contributed to the development of the WHO/ UNICEF community component of the integrated management of childhood illness (IMCI) that emphasises: improving partnerships between health facilities and the communities they serve; increasing appropriate and accessible health care and information from community-based providers, and integrating promotion of key family practices critical for child health and nutrition (CORE Group, 2009).

Positive psychology emphasises the importance of the environment in its totality in shaping individual wellbeing and flourishing. Individuals need a supportive environment to grow, develop, and thrive – an environment that provides opportunities for social and meaningful connection, focuses on and cultivates individuals' strengths, creates opportunities for individuals to achieve their full potential, and is a place to feel safe and peaceful. Research indicates that positive relationships and a sense of belonging contribute significantly to overall wellbeing and resilience (Lambert et al., 2013; Lyons et al., 2016; Nowicki, 2008). Positive environments support individuals' autonomy and provide opportunities for mastery and growth (De-Juanas et al., 2020; Ryff & Keyes, 1995). Environments that foster a sense of autonomy, competence, and mastery empower individuals to pursue their goals and engage in meaningful activities (Ryff & Keyes, 1995), as both individual and environmental factors interact to shape wellbeing and advocate for interventions and policies that enhance wellbeing.

However, the environments we have discussed are not separate or mutually exclusive. We chose the physical, built, cultural, and social environments as illustrative examples, but each intersects, overlaps, and connects with the other. For example, the legal environment within these other environments contributes to our conditions of justice which are inextricably linked with wellbeing: "Optimal conditions of justice, suboptimal conditions of justice, vulnerable conditions of injustice, and persisting conditions of injustice lead to thriving, coping, confronting, and suffering, respectively" (Prilleltensky, 2012). It is these interactions, connections, relationships, or interfacing of people and the environments that we now explore further.

## POSITIVE HEALTH AND THE ENVIRONMENT

Positive health embraces positive psychology and lifestyle medicine interventions, but proposes that combining these interventions will improve the lifestyle behavioural outcomes of happier and healthier people. Additionally, the importance of all ecosystems and their connection to wellbeing is recognised explicitly and a more integrated approach to interventions is proposed – making that connection between the different elements of the system – to flourish in life. For example, positive health recognises that taking a walk in nature or engaging in the creative arts, for example, improve wellbeing through physical, physiological, and psychological processes. However, there is also the acknowledgement that environmental exposures do not impact everyone equally, that we are also continuously changing the environment by being in it, and that there are multiple levels beyond the individual level through which these processes occur. An environmental positive health intervention would take a more systemic approach, such as encouraging walks in nature, but recognising we live in a shared environment and that to achieve this a collaborative approach that supports the creation of walking spaces in a biodiverse built environment will encourage flourishing of all. It is also about empowering people with the ability to adapt, self-manage, and develop resilience on that journey to flourishing.

Some examples of positive interventions that embrace a holistic and systemic approach in practice include:

**Modelling the connections**: Vodovotz et al. (2024) argue that when individuals experience stress, it can lead to chronic inflammation and problems with thinking. This can spread to entire populations through the following steps:

- Stress and inflammation can pass from one person to many in a population.
- If many people in a population have chronic inflammation, it can affect how everyone makes decisions and behaves.
- This can make it harder for the population to deal with the original stress.
- The problems feed off each other, creating a big problem that affects society and even the environment on a global scale.

The increased connectivity in the world, such as social media, fuels the spread. They present a mathematical model that suggests the need for more systems, a coordinated and inter-disciplinary approach to interventions, and research around these interventions. These could be termed positive health interventions. One example is lifestyle changes in terms of nutrition, exercise, and reduced exposure to stressful online content, but with interventions at a broader level around constructing calm public spaces and education around societal norms and regulations in mitigating the risk of societal inflammation. Overall, a more systems approach to dealing with stress is argued for.

**System approaches to policies**: An example of this is proposed by Sallis and colleagues (Sallis et al., 2016) in terms of land use and transport policies. Land-use and transport policies globally contribute to widespread health issues, including injuries and non–communicable diseases due to factors like traffic exposure, noise, and air pollution. Urban planning often overlooks these health impacts, despite evidence suggesting that integrating health considerations could address many common health problems. They advocate for urban and transport planning decisions to prioritise compact, mixed-use designs that promote walking, cycling, and public transport over private vehicles. By emphasising active transport and sustainable urban mobility, cities can improve population health and sustainability in the long term.

**Nature-based solutions**: The Connecting Nature project (Collier et al., 2023) uses a three-stage process to promote nature-based solutions in cities. This involves seven key activity areas: technical solutions, governance, financing, nature-based businesses, co-production, monitoring, and impact assessment. The framework helps overcome barriers to implementing these solutions through a collaborative, iterative, and reflective approach. Initially the focus was on nature-inspired innovations – so, beneficial to the environment but also creating business opportunities. Currently the research is around reconnecting people with the wild especially through biodiversity in urban areas with preliminary findings suggesting lifestyle behavioural changes and increased wellbeing.

## A RELATIONAL APPROACH TO WELLBEING

Bilbao-Nieva and Meyer (2024) suggest that we look at relational approaches to wellbeing, where we see wellbeing as something shaped by connections between people and their surroundings, rather than centred on the individual. In this way wellbeing isn't seen as a fixed state or something that can be attained by or within individuals, but as something that emerges from the interactions and dynamics of communities and their surroundings. This perspective shifts the focus from individuals to the connections or relationships between them, highlighting the complex and continuously changing nature of wellbeing. Instead of focusing solely on how individuals think or feel, these approaches look at the relationships people have with one another and the environments they live in. Adopting this approach assists in understanding the very personal nature of wellbeing.

For example, one of the dimensions of wellbeing from the work of Ryff and Keyes (1995) is mastery of the environment – reflecting an individual's capacity to effectively navigate, adapt to, and shape their environment in ways that promote personal growth, satisfaction, and wellbeing. However, environmental mastery overlaps with the other dimensions of wellbeing and autonomy, personal growth, positive relations with others, purpose in life and self-acceptance. These dimensions are important in their own right, but also how they interact with the environment. However, this thinking is centred around the individual, whereas Bilbao-Nieva and Meyer (2024) propose looking at wellbeing as arising from the relationship or connection to our environment, not as a result. Barad (Barad, 2003, 2007), in fact, questions the idea of individuals as separate from everything else, but as interacting with, the environment. When we think about wellbeing in this way, we consider how it is connected to everything around us, not just something only people experience.

This way of thinking fits in with New Materialism – a way of thinking that sees humans as part of and connected to the world around us and focuses on breaking down the differences between humans and everything else in the natural world with an emphasis on equal attention to humans and nonhumans (Gamble et al., 2019). This perspective recognises that our actions physically change things around and within us. In this view, everything is always changing, and no one thing starts it all. Barad uses the term intra-action ("the mutual constitution of entangled agencies" 2007, p. 33) rather than interaction to describe the relationship between humans and the material world where everything is mixed up together – humans and the material world affect each other and change together.

A relativist view is not opposed to the views described above and our connections with the environment, but offers another lens to more deeply understand the complexity of this entangled relationship. To illustrate this, Bilbao-Nieva and Meyer (2024) give an account of a young girl's role in, and process of, caring for her sister, their relationship and entanglement within the house's structure, the weather, and other resources from which wellbeing emerged. It illustrates how wellbeing is part of a bigger picture involving people, materiality, and their surroundings. It emphasises that wellbeing does not require ideal conditions to happen; instead, it can be understood as an ever-changing process. This story serves as an example of why we should be interested in understanding the ongoing process of wellbeing, which goes beyond feelings or thoughts.

### Antonia and moments of wellbeing

*Antonia is a 15-year-old girl living in the rugged beauty of Chilean Patagonia. She shares a small home with her mother and older sister, who is 18 and has a physical disability that prevents her from walking. When asked about her wellbeing, Antonia begins by talking about the good and the bad in her life. "What is good about home is that the three of us live together", she says, her voice tinged with a mix of pride and weariness. Despite the challenges, she treasures the moments they spend together. They cook, bake, listen to music, and watch television. However, these activities are rare treats because their mother works full-time and is often away from home.*

*Antonia's sister's disability requires constant care, and Antonia has taken on the role of her primary caregiver. This responsibility weighs heavily on her young shoulders. Her sister can be moody and irritable, and when she is cranky, it affects the entire family and the home environment. "She gets irritable. She is used to having everything as she likes. Or that we are always making her company", Antonia explains. "It must be frustrating not to be able to do certain things. Maybe this is the way she has for venting."*

*Antonia then shares a concrete example of what wellbeing means to her, a situation that diverges from traditional definitions of the term. She describes a typical day when her mother had to leave for work at 2 pm and her sister was in pain. The previous evening, her mother planned to bathe her sister but couldn't because Antonia forgot to turn on the heater. The house needs to be warm for her sister's bath, so Antonia promised to take care of it the next day. "I waited until 3 pm to bathe her because it was sunnier", Antonia recounts. "The house was warmer when I started the heater. Then I bathed her. Her legs were in pain. It was hard, but I bathed her. And she was still in pain."*

*Despite the difficulty, Antonia did not stop there. She cooked some milanesas (a variation of schnitzel) to have with tea, a simple comfort food. Then she suggested they watch movies together. "The Little Mermaid, Cinderella, the kind of things she likes", Antonia says, a small smile breaking through her serious expression. "And then she was calmed."*

*This, to Antonia, is a moment of wellbeing. It is not about grand gestures or moments of perfect happiness. It is about the small, everyday acts of care and love that she provides for her sister. It is about creating a sense of comfort and normalcy in a life that is anything but.*

*Antonia's story highlights a different understanding of wellbeing. It is rarely told but deeply significant. Her wellbeing is not defined by her own comfort or ease but by the moments when she can bring relief and happiness to her sister. It is the warmth of the house after the heater has been turned on, the simple meal shared over tea, and the familiar, comforting stories of animated princesses. Her story is a powerful reminder that wellbeing can be found in the quiet acts of love and care we give to those we cherish.*

Based on Antonio's story in Bibao-Nieva (2022) and Bilbao-Nieva et al. (2024).

In assessing the *Wakakosha* intervention mentioned above, this relational perspective of wellbeing helps explain our findings better. What emerged from our study were several cultural and contextual insights into positive health, namely the culture surrounding discussing feelings and emotions, spirituality, and individual versus collective agency (Ferris France et al., 2023). As with other sub-Saharan African countries, men culturally find it difficult to express emotions and feelings freely due to societal norms. However, after the intervention they reported the ability to do so. Spirituality had both positive effects, such as God giving you only what you have the strength to handle, and negative effects, such as punishment for wrongdoing of the past, on wellbeing. The intervention helped participants make sense of these thoughts and beliefs in relation to who they were and their actions. Additionally, what emerged was a strong collectivist culture where the wellbeing of others is as important, if not more, than your own – in fact, it was hard for participants to separate the two. So wellbeing was embedded in the connections in the different levels within the social and cultural environments – the cultural acceptability of men sharing feelings, the importance of spirituality and individual versus interdependent cultures. This in some way can be explained in positive psychology through altruism (Batson et al., 2002) and compassion (Gilbert, 2010), but as Wong notes, "there are cultural differences in the balancing act between me and we. ... we need to emphasise positive motivations, processes, activities, and outcomes for both individuals and groups" (2011, p. 72). A relativist approach to wellbeing captures and embraces this complexity well.

## SUMMARY

The relationship between our environment and wellbeing is dynamic and influenced by relationships; it can reshape priorities, policies, and social norms and how we design and implement positive health interventions. Wellbeing is not an isolated process pertaining to an individual, nor is it a fixed state. In other words, wellbeing is a journey and not a destination. Just like our environment, wellbeing is continuously changing and is different for everyone. A relativist approach to wellbeing enables the capturing of both positive and negative states of health, how words, actions, beliefs, and structures are important, why collectivist and individual wellbeing are difficult to disentangle in some cultures and how spirituality and traditional knowledge hold significance in these connections. The proposed relativist approach to wellbeing supports environmental sustainability, social justice, and multi-level analysis of wellbeing beyond the individual (Bilbao-Nieva & Meyer, 2024; Prilleltensky, 2012). Such an approach also offers valuable insights into understanding wellbeing as dynamic and fluid, shaped by ongoing interactions and relationships and can advance our understanding of the diversity of wellbeing and its implications for individuals and societies. It rebalances the view of wellbeing as an overall state of flourishing and not just wellbeing of the individual in the environment they live in. Equal importance to and emphasis on the connection of the individual, the community, the society, and fundamentally the planet is given, where individual wellbeing is not prioritised over environmental wellbeing – they cannot be treated separately as they are intra-connected.

Overall, we can think of wellbeing like a shape-shifting puzzle. This puzzle does not have one fixed form but comes in various shapes and sizes, depending on how we interact with the world. These interactions, like the pieces of a puzzle, fit together to create our perception and experience of wellbeing, and relationship with our environment. And, just like a puzzle, it's always evolving, with new pieces being added and rearranged over time. So, our understanding and approach to wellbeing are constantly changing too, influenced by the ongoing interactions between us and our environment.

# REFERENCES

Adelson, E., Maitra, S., & Nastasi, B. K. (2017). Informing sexual health intervention development in India: Perspectives of daughters, mothers, and service providers in Mumbai. *International Journal of School & Educational Psychology*, 5(3), 167–177. https://doi.org/10.1080/21683603.2016.1276814

Adelson, E., Nastasi, B. K., Maitra, S., Ballal, D., & Rajan, L. (2016). Sexual health, gender roles, and psychological well-being: Voices of female adolescents from urban slums of India. In B. K. Nastasi & A. P. Borja (Eds.), *International handbook of psychological well-being in children and adolescents: Bridging the gaps between theory, research, and practice* (pp. 79–96). Springer New York. https://doi.org/10.1007/978-1-4939-2833-0_6

Ahmed, S. (2010). *The promise of happiness*. Duke University Press. https://doi.org/10.1215/9780822392781

Bam, J. (2021). *Ausi told me: Why Cape herstoriographies matter*. Jacana Media. https://books.google.ie/books?id=faLyzgEACAAJ

Barad, K. (2003). Posthumanist performativity: Toward an understanding of how matter comes to matter. *Signs: Journal of Women in Culture and Society*, 28(3), 473–494. www.journals.uchicago.edu/doi/10.1086/345321

Barad, K. (2007). *Meeting the universe halfway: Quantum physics and the entanglement of matter and meaning*. Duke University Press.

Batson, C. D., Ahmad, N., Lishner, D. A., & Tsan, J.-A. (2002). Empathy and altruism. In C. R. Snyder & S. J. Lopez (Eds.), *Handbook of positive psychology* (pp. 485–498). Oxford University Press.

Baur, J. W., Gómez, E., & Tynon, J. F. (2013). Urban nature parks and neighborhood social health in Portland, Oregon. *Journal of Park & Recreation Administration*, 31(4), 23–44.

Berman, M. G., Kross, E., Krpan, K. M., Askren, M. K., Burson, A., Deldin, P. J., Kaplan, S., Sherdell, L., Gotlib, I. H., & Jonides, J. (2012). Interacting with nature improves cognition and affect for individuals with depression. *Journal of Affective Disorders*, 140(3), 300–305. https://doi.org/10.1016/j.jad.2012.03.012

Bilbao-Nieva, M. I. (2022). *Discourses of well-being of adolescent girls living in Patagonia, Chile*. Michigan State University.

Bilbao-Nieva, M., & Meyer, A. (2024). Contributions of Barad's new materialism to well-being research. *The Qualitative Report*, 29(4), 898–914.

Blackie, S. (2016). *If women rose rooted: A life-changing journey to authenticity and belonging*. September Publishing. https://books.google.ie/books?id=B_w2EAAAQBAJ

Bronfenbrenner, U. (1979). *The ecology of human development*. Harvard University Press.

Brown, G., Reeders, D., Cogle, A., Allan, B., Howard, C., Rule, J., Chong, S., & Gleeson, D. (2022). Tackling structural stigma: A systems perspective. *Journal of the International AIDS Society*, *25*, e25924.

Burke, J., & Arslan, G. (2020). Positive education and school psychology during COVID-19 pandemic. *Journal of Positive Psychology and Wellbeing*, *4*(2), 137–139.

Burke, J., Dunne, P., Byrne, E., & O'Boyle, C. (2024). Ch 4: Positive physical health. In *Positive health: The basics*. Routledge.

Byrne, E., & Gregory, J. (2007). Co-constructing local meanings for child health indicators in community-based information systems: The UThukela District Child Survival Project in KwaZulu-Natal. *International Journal of Medical Informatics*, *76 Suppl 1*, S78–88. https://doi.org/10.1016/j.ijmedinf.2006.05.018

Cabanas, E., & Illouz, E. (2019). *Happycracia. Cómo la ciencia y la industria de la felicidad controlan nuestras vidas*. Ediciones Paidós.

Carreno, D. F., Eisenbeck, N., Greville, J., & Wong, P. T. P. (2023). Cross-Cultural psychometric analysis of the mature happiness scale-revised: Mature happiness, psychological inflexibility, and the PERMA model. *Journal of Happiness Studies*, *24*(3), 1075–1099. https://doi.org/10.1007/s10902-023-00633-7

Chirico, F. (2016). Spiritual wellbeing in the 21st century: It's time to review the current WHO's health definition. *Journal of Health and Social Sciences*, *1*(1), 11–16.

Collier, M. J., Frantzeskaki, N., Connop, S., Dick, G., Dumitru, A., Dziubała, A., Fletcher, I., Georgiou, P., Hölscher, K., Kooijman, E., Lodder, M., Madajczyk, N., McQuaid, S., Nash, C., Osipiuk, A., Quartier, M., Reil, A., Rhodes, M.-L., Rizzi, D., Vandergert, P., Sijpe, K. V. D., Vos, P., & Xidous, D. (2023). An integrated process for planning, delivery, and stewardship of urban nature-based solutions: The Connecting Nature Framework. *Nature-Based Solutions*, *3*, 100060. https://doi.org/10.1016/j.nbsj.2023.100060

CORE Group. (2009). *Community-based Integrated Management of Childhood Illness Policy Guidance*. www.fsnnetwork.org/resource/community-based-integrated-management-childhood-illnesses-c-imci-program-guidance

Dambi, J. M., Cowan, F. M., Martin, F., Sibanda, S., Simms, V., Willis, N., Bernays, S., & Mavhu, W. (2022). Conceptualisation and psychometric evaluation of positive psychological outcome measures used in adolescents and young adults living with HIV: A mixed scoping and systematic review protocol. *BMJ Open*, *12*(9), e066129. https://doi.org/10.1136/bmjopen-2022-066129

De-Juanas, Á., Bernal Romero, T., & Goig, R. (2020). The relationship between psychological wellbeing and autonomy in young people according to age. *Frontiers in Psychology*, *11*, 559976.

Dockx, Y., Bijnens, E. M., Luyten, L., Peusens, M., Provost, E., Rasking, L., Sleurs, H., Hogervorst, J., Plusquin, M., Casas, L., & Nawrot, T. S. (2022). Early life exposure to residential green space impacts cognitive functioning in children aged 4 to 6 years. *Environ Int*, *161*, 107094. https://doi.org/10.1016/j.envint.2022.107094

Earth Horizon (2018, 7 February). *Tackling the obesity crisis in Ireland with Donal O'Shea*. https://youtu.be/_Jppo0Mhqek?si=xiDcVCgrM7a_hauY

Ferguson, S. T. M., Murtagh, B., & Ellis, G. (2016). *Understanding rural walkability: The PASTORAL study in Northern Ireland* (Doctoral thesis, Queen's University Belfast).

Ferris France, N., Byrne, E., Nyamwanza, O., Munatsi, V., Willis, N., Conroy, R., Vumbunu, S., Chinembiri, M., Maedziso, S., Katsande, M. A., Dongo, T. A., Crehan, E., & Mavhu, W. (2023). Wakakosha "You are Worth it": reported impact of a community-based, peer-led HIV self-stigma intervention to improve self-worth and wellbeing among young people living with HIV in Zimbabwe [Original Research]. *Frontiers in Public Health*, *11*. https://doi.org/10.3389/fpubh.2023.1235150

Gamble, C. N., Hanan, J. S., & Nail, T. (2019). What is new materialism? *Angelaki*, *24*(6), 111–134. https://doi.org/10.1080/0969725X.2019.1684704

Gilbert, P. (2010). *The compassionate mind: A new approach to life's challenges*. New Harbinger Publications. https://books.google.ie/books?id=krNPL6xCVL0C

Gruber, J., Mauss, I. B., & Tamir, M. (2011). A dark side of happiness? How, when, and why happiness is not always good. *Perspectives on Psychological Science*, *6*(3), 222–233.

Guse, T. (2022). Positive psychological interventions in African contexts: A scoping review. In L. Schutte, T. Guse, & M. P. Wissing (Eds.), *Embracing wellbeing in diverse African contexts: Research perspectives* (pp. 375–397). Springer International Publishing. https://doi.org/10.1007/978-3-030-85924-4_16

Ibeneme, S., Eni, G., Ezuma, A., & Fortwengel, G. (2017). Roads to health in developing countries: Understanding the intersection of culture and healing. *Current Therapeutic Research*, *86*, 13–18. https://doi.org/10.1016/j.curtheres.2017.03.001

Ideno, Y., Hayashi, K., Abe, Y., Ueda, K., Iso, H., Noda, M., Lee, J. S., & Suzuki, S. (2017). Blood pressure-lowering effect of Shinrin-yoku (Forest bathing): A systematic review and meta-analysis. *BMC Complementary and Alternative Medicine*, *17*(1), 409. https://doi.org/10.1186/s12906-017-1912-z

Keenan, R., Lumber, R., Richardson, M., & Sheffield, D. (2021). Three good things in nature: A nature-based positive psychological intervention to improve mood and well-being for depression and anxiety. *Journal of Public Mental Health*, *20*, 243–250. https://doi.org/s://doi.org/10.1108/jpmh-02-2021-0029

Lai, L. C.-H. (2022). The relative importance of self-esteem and collective self-esteem to subjective wellbeing: A study of Hong Kong Chinese and Australian Chinese. *Research Developments in Arts and Social Studies*, 7, 33–45.

Lambert, N. M., Stillman, T. F., Hicks, J. A., Kamble, S., Baumeister, R. F., & Fincham, F. D. (2013). To belong is to matter: Sense of belonging enhances meaning in life. *Personality and Social Psychology Bulletin*, *39*(11), 1418–1427. https://doi.org/10.1177/0146167213499186

Leddy, T. (2015). Experience of awe: An expansive approach to everyday aesthetics. *Contemporary Aesthetics (Journal Archive)*, *13*(1), 8.

Lomas, T. (2016). Towards a positive cross-cultural lexicography: Enriching our emotional landscape through 216 "untranslatable" words pertaining to wellbeing. *The Journal of Positive Psychology*, *11*(5), 546–558. https://doi.org/10.1080/17439760.2015.1127993

Lomas, T. (2021). Towards a cross-cultural lexical map of wellbeing. *The Journal of Positive Psychology*, *16*(5), 622–639. https://doi.org/10.1080/17439760.2020.1791944

Louv, R. (2008). *Last child in the woods: Saving our children from nature-deficit disorder*. Algonquin Books. https://books.google.ie/books?id=_J8ymvTQz8kC

Løvoll, H. S., Sæther, K.-W., & Graves, M. (2020). Feeling at home in the wilderness: Environmental conditions, wellbeing and aesthetic experience. *Frontiers in Psychology*, *11*, 501609.

Lyons, A., Fletcher, G., Farmer, J., Kenny, A., Bourke, L., Carra, K., & Bariola, E. (2016). Participation in rural community groups and links with psychological wellbeing and resilience: A cross-sectional community-based study. *BMC Psychology*, *4*, 1–10.

Markus, H., & Kitayama, S. (1991). Culture and the self: Implications for cognition, emotion, and motivation. *Psychological Review*, *98*, 224–253.

Mastandrea, S., Fagioli, S., & Biasi, V. (2019). Art and psychological wellbeing: Linking the brain to the aesthetic emotion. *Frontiers in Psychology*, *10*, 430007.

Muthukrishna, M., Bell, A. V., Henrich, J., Curtin, C. M., Gedranovich, A., McInerney, J., & Thue, B. (2020). Beyond western, educated, industrial, rich, and democratic (WEIRD) psychology: Measuring and mapping scales of cultural and psychological distance. *Psychological Science*, *31*(6), 678–701. https://doi.org/10.1177/0956797620916782

Nerstad, C. G. L., Wong, S. I., & Richardsen, A. M. (2019). Can engagement go awry and lead to burnout? The moderating role of the perceived motivational climate. *International Journal of Environmental Research and Public Health*, *16*(11). https://doi.org/10.3390/ijerph16111979

Nowicki, A. (2008). Self-efficacy, sense of belonging and social support as predictors of resilience in adolescents. Unpublished thesis.

O'Boyle, C. A., Lianov, L., Burke, J., Frates, B., & Boniwell, I. (2024). Positive health: An emerging new construct. In J. Burke, I. Boniwell, B. Frates, L. Lianov, & C. A. O'Boyle (Eds.), *LMRoutledge international handbook of positive health sciences*. Routledge.

Park, B. J., Tsunetsugu, Y., Kasetani, T., Kagawa, T., & Miyazaki, Y. (2010). The physiological effects of Shinrin-yoku (taking in the forest atmosphere or forest bathing): Evidence from field experiments in 24 forests across Japan. *Environmental Health and Preventive Medicine*, *15*(1), 18–26. https://doi.org/10.1007/s12199-009-0086-9

Passmore, H.-A., & Holder, M. D. (2017). Noticing nature: Individual and social benefits of a two-week intervention. *The Journal of Positive Psychology*, *12*(6), 537–546. https://doi.org/10.1080/17439760.2016.1221126

Passmore, H.-A., Yang, Y., & Sabine, S. (2022). An extended replication study of the well-being intervention, the noticing nature intervention (NNI). *Journal of Happiness Studies*, *23*(6), 2663–2683. https://doi.org/10.1007/s10902-022-00516-3

Peterson, C., Park, N., & Sweeney, P. J. (2008). Group well-being: Morale from a positive psychology perspective. *Applied Psychology*, *57*(s1), 19–36. https://doi.org/10.1111/j.1464-0597.2008.00352.x

Prilleltensky, I. (2012). Wellness as fairness. *American Journal of Community Psychology*, *49*(1–2), 1–21. https://doi.org/10.1007/s10464-011-9448-8

Prinsloo, C. D., Greeff, M., Kruger, A., & Ellis, S. (2016). Psychosocial wellbeing of people living with HIV and the community before and after a HIV stigma-reduction community "hub" network intervention. *African Journal of AIDS Research*, *15*, 261–271.

Raworth, K. (2017). *Doughnut economics: Seven ways to think like a 21st-century economist*. Chelsea Green Publishing. https://books.google.ie/books?id=SUYtDgAAQBAJ

Ryff, C. D. (2022). Positive psychology: Looking back and looking forward [systematic review]. *Frontiers in Psychology*, *13*. https://doi.org/10.3389/fpsyg.2022.840062

Ryff, C. D., & Keyes, C. L. M. (1995). The structure of psychological wellbeing revisited. *Journal of Personality and Social Psychology*, *69*(4), 719.

Sagner, M., Egger, E., Binns, A., & Rossner, S. (2017). *LM: Lifestyle, the environment and preventive medicine in health and disease* (3rd ed.). Academic Press.

Sallis, J. F., Bull, F., Burdett, R., Frank, L. D., Griffiths, P., Giles-Corti, B., & Stevenson, M. (2016). Use of science to guide city planning policy and practice: How to achieve healthy and sustainable future cities. *Lancet*, *388*(10062), 2936–2947. https://doi.org/10.1016/s0140-6736(16)30068-x

Selhub, E. M., & Logan, A. C. (2012). *Your brain on nature: The science of nature's influence on your health, happiness and vitality*. John Wiley & Sons.

Seligman, M. E., & Csikszentmihalyi, M. (2000). *Positive psychology: An introduction* (Vol. 55). American Psychological Association.

Smit, W., Hancock, T., Kumaresen, J., Santos-Burgoa, C., Sánchez-Kobashi Meneses, R., Friel, S., Smit, W., Hancock, T., Kumaresen, J., Santos-Burgoa, C., Sánchez-Kobashi Meneses, R., & Friel, S. (2011). Toward a research and action agenda on urban planning/design and health equity in cities in low and middle-income countries. *Journal of Urban Health, 88*(5), 875–885. https://doi.org/10.1007/s11524-011-9605-2

Stangl, A. L., Lloyd, J. K., Brady, L. M., Holland, C. E., & Baral, S. (2013). A systematic review of interventions to reduce HIV-related stigma and discrimination from 2002 to 2013: How far have we come? *Journal of the International AIDS Society, 16*, 18734.

Tam, K.-P., Lau, H. P. B., & Jiang, D. (2012). Culture and subjective wellbeing: A dynamic constructivist view. *Journal of Cross-Cultural Psychology, 43*(1), 23–31.

van den Berg, A. E., Maas, J., Verheij, R. A., & Groenewegen, P. P. (2010). Green space as a buffer between stressful life events and health. *Social Science and Medicine, 70*(8), 1203–1210. https://doi.org/10.1016/j.socscimed.2010.01.002

Vodovotz, Y., Arciero, J., Verschure, P. F. M. J., & Katz, D. L. (2024). A multiscale inflammatory map: Linking individual stress to societal dysfunction [Frontiers in Science Lead Article]. *Frontiers in Science, 1.* https://doi.org/10.3389/fsci.2023.1239462

Wells, N. M., & Evans, G. W. (2003). Nearby nature: A buffer of life stress among rural children. *Environment and Behavior, 35*(3), 311–330. https://doi.org/10.1177/0013916503035003001

Wen, Y., Yan, Q., Pan, Y., Gu, X., & Liu, Y. (2019). Medical empirical research on forest bathing (Shinrin-yoku): A systematic review. *Environmental Health and Preventive Medicine, 24*(1), 70. https://doi.org/10.1186/s12199-019-0822-8

White, M. P., Alcock, I., Wheeler, B. W., & Depledge, M. H. (2013). Would you be happier living in a greener urban area? A fixed-effects analysis of panel data. *Psychological Science, 24*(6), 920–928. https://doi.org/10.1177/0956797612464659

Wong, P. T. P. (2011). Positive psychology 2.0: Towards a balanced interactive model of the good life. *Canadian Psychology/Psychologie canadienne, 52*(2), 69–81.

# THE FUTURE OF POSITIVE HEALTH

Positive health, a novel and exciting field is the integration of positive psychology research with lifestyle medicine. In this book, we aimed to present our unique perspective on positive health from the Royal College of Surgeons in Ireland (RCSI), University of Medicine and Health Sciences. Our viewpoint stands out due to its innovative grounding in lifestyle medicine – a rigorously researched field focused on interventions designed to reduce noncommunicable diseases, which account for 73% of global deaths annually; also, due to combining lifestyle medicine with positive psychology research exploring the good life.

While lifestyle medicine is comprehensive, addressing factors such as diet, exercise, and stress management, it traditionally does not incorporate the principles of positive psychology. Positive psychology, the science of optimal human functioning, goes beyond the basic concept of wellbeing. It posits that a strong foundation of wellbeing can significantly enhance one's ability to adopt and maintain healthy lifestyle choices.

Positive health emerged from the necessity to blend the principles of positive psychology, salutogenesis theories, and health psychology with lifestyle medicine to maximise its impact on health outcomes. Health professionals, researchers, and policymakers are crucial in this integration process. Salutogenesis, which focuses on factors that support human health and wellbeing rather than on factors that cause disease, complements the aims of lifestyle medicine and positive psychology.

We are in the early stages of exploring and implementing positive health, but we are optimistic about its potential. We hope that this

DOI: 10.4324/9781003457169-7

integrated approach will reduce the burden of non-communicable diseases and promote a holistic sense of wellbeing, ultimately leading to better health outcomes and an enriched quality of life.

## FUTURE DIRECTIONS FOR RESEARCHERS

To advance the field of positive health, researchers can focus on several key areas to integrate lifestyle medicine and positive psychology effectively, ensuring a comprehensive approach to positive health and wellbeing. Here are some steps researchers can take:

### INTERDISCIPLINARY COLLABORATION

Researchers from diverse fields such as psychology, medicine, public health, and sociology should collaborate to develop a unified framework for positive health. This interdisciplinary approach can lead to a more comprehensive understanding of health and wellbeing using the positive psychology perspective and design studies that explore how lifestyle interventions and positive psychological practices can be combined to enhance health outcomes.

### LONGITUDINAL STUDIES

Conducting long-term studies will provide valuable insights into the sustained effects of integrated positive health interventions. These studies can track participants over several years to understand how combining lifestyle medicine and positive psychology impacts their health, wellbeing, and longevity.

### DEVELOPMENT OF COMPREHENSIVE INTERVENTIONS

Designing and testing comprehensive interventions that incorporate elements of lifestyle medicine (such as healthy eating, physical activity, and stress management) and positive psychology (including gratitude practices, resilience training, and strengths-based approaches). For instance, a comprehensive intervention could involve a structured exercise programme and mindfulness and wellbeing training. Researchers should evaluate the effectiveness of these combined interventions through randomised controlled trials and mediating and moderating factors for their effectiveness. They could also expand their methodologies beyond the quantitative research and explore the impact of positive health interventions using qualitative research designs.

### TECHNOLOGY INTEGRATION

Applying technology such as artificial intelligence, mobile (smartphone) applications (apps), wearable devices, and telehealth platforms to deliver and monitor positive health interventions. For example, a mobile app could deliver daily mindfulness exercises and track the user's progress. Technology can facilitate real-time data collection, provide personalised feedback, and enhance engagement with health-promoting activities.

### PATIENTS AND PUBLIC INVOLVEMENT RESEARCH

Engaging in community-based participatory research to understand different populations' unique needs and challenges. This research involves active participation from community members, who provide valuable insights and help tailor interventions to be culturally relevant and more effective in promoting positive health.

### METRICS AND ASSESSMENT TOOLS

Developing and validating comprehensive assessment tools measuring lifestyle and psychological factors contributing to positive health. These tools should capture the multi-dimensional nature of health and wellbeing, providing a holistic view of an individual's health status.

## FUTURE DIRECTIONS FOR HEALTHCARE

### EDUCATION AND TRAINING

Developing educational programmes and training modules for healthcare providers to integrate positive health principles into their practice. Training could cover both the theoretical and practical aspects of positive health and Positive Psychology, equipping professionals with the skills to support their patients holistically.

## POLICY ADVOCACY

Advocating for policies that support the integration of positive health into healthcare systems. Researchers can work with policymakers to promote funding for positive health initiatives, create supportive environments for healthy living, and implement community-based programmes that emphasise physical and psychological wellbeing.

## PUBLIC AWARENESS CAMPAIGNS

Increasing public awareness about the importance of positive health through campaigns highlighting the benefits of integrating lifestyle medicine and positive psychology. By engaging with these campaigns, everyone can play a crucial role in educating and motivating people to adopt healthier lifestyles and positive psychological practices, thereby promoting positive health.

# FUTURE DIRECTIONS FOR EVERY PERSON WHO HOPES TO LIVE A GOOD LIFE

Imagine a world where the principles of positive health, a wholistic approach encompassing physical, mental, and social wellbeing, are integrated into society, impacting every stage of life and every aspect of daily living. In this world, everyone would be equipped with the knowledge and tools to enhance their health and wellbeing, leading to a thriving, healthier global community. Here is our vision of what the world will look like if we integrate positive health into our daily lives.

## BIRTH

From the moment a baby is born, positive health will become a foundation for children and their parents. Soon-to-be mothers will be educated on how to look after their bodies and mind during pregnancy and when giving birth to their children. New mothers will receive the support of a positive health coach, who will work closely with them to navigate the challenges of early motherhood. This support will include strategies such as a perinatal wellbeing programme that spans from perinatal to postnatal engagement, mindfulness exercises to boost mental health, postnatal yoga and positive health activities to prevent postnatal depression, and create a joyful, nurturing environment for the baby. Fathers and other caregivers will also be included in this support network, ensuring the whole family benefits from positive health principles.

## EMPOWERING YOUNG MINDS

Educational institutions will play a crucial role in fostering positive health from a young age. Schools will incorporate positive health education into their curricula, teaching children about the importance of a balanced diet, regular exercise, and mental resilience. Programmes on positive health will help students understand and apply concepts such as mindfulness, optimism, good nutrition and strengths-based development.

Young people learn to thrive academically and personally, equipped with the skills to manage stress, build strong relationships, and confidently pursue their goals. In the future, they will experience lower levels of non-communicable diseases, such as obesity, stroke, or other chronic diseases of lifestyle. Positive health's foundation will prepare them for adulthood's challenges, contributing to a society where psychological flourishing is the norm.

## FLOURISHING WORKPLACES

As these children grow and eventually enter the workforce, they find that positive health will be an integral part of their professional lives. Workplaces across the globe will offer comprehensive positive health programmes designed to reduce the incidence of non-communicable diseases and promote mental wellbeing. These programmes will include regular physical activity sessions, healthy eating workshops, advice on getting healthy sleep, stress management techniques, and positive psychology practices such as gratitude journaling and resilience training. Technology will play a crucial role in these initiatives, providing personalised health recommendations, tracking progress, and ensuring data privacy and security.

Employers will recognise that a healthy, happy workforce is more productive and innovative. Employees will be encouraged to take care of their physical health through lifestyle medicine while nurturing their mental health with positive psychology tools.

This wholistic approach will improves employees' wellbeing and create a workplace culture where people feel valued, supported, and motivated to excel, leading to increased productivity and job satisfaction. Due to collective efforts, prevention will overtake the cure approaches, allowing the populations to live flourishing and healthy lives.

### HEALING HANDS, POSITIVE HEARTS

Doctors and healthcare professionals will seamlessly integrate positive health into their practice alongside traditional medical approaches in hospitals and medical centres. Patients will receive holistic care that addresses their physical ailments and their mental and emotional wellbeing. They will be empowered to take care of their health and wellbeing. Positive health tools, such as meditation-based practices, stress reduction techniques, lifestyle medicine, and nature-based interventions, will be prescribed alongside medications, surgeries, and treatments. This comprehensive approach will empower patients to actively participate in their healing journey and maintain healthy lifestyle choices long after they leave the hospital. Subsequently, the incidence of non-communicable diseases will continue to decrease year on year, and so will the statistics for mental health issues.

### THRIVING COMMUNITIES, VIBRANT LIVES

Communities will emerge as vibrant wellbeing hubs, where positive health will become part of their daily life. Local leaders, grassroots organisations, and community members will unite to create environments that support health and happiness. Natural resources like forests, parks, and green spaces will become essential to community wellbeing. Nature-prescribing programmes will encourage individuals to reconnect with the healing power of the outdoors, promoting physical activity, mental rejuvenation, and a deep connection to the world around them. These initiatives will respect and celebrate the diversity of cultural and social practices, integrating positive health in an inclusive way.

At the heart of this vision are empowered individuals who will recognise their innate capacity to shape their health and wellbeing.

People of all ages and backgrounds will embrace positive health as a lifelong journey of self-discovery, growth, and empowerment. They will cultivate resilience, optimism, and a sense of purpose that fuels their pursuit of wellbeing in every aspect of their lives. Through education, support, and community engagement, individuals will harness the transformative power of positive health to overcome challenges, pursue their passions, and live lives filled with meaning and fulfilment.

## A GLOBAL MOVEMENT, A BETTER WORLD

Positive health will become a global movement for positive change as it spreads its wings and takes flight. Governments, policymakers, and international organisations prioritise wellbeing as a fundamental human right and integrate positive health into public health initiatives, education systems, and social policies. The ripple effects of this movement will be felt far and wide as societies worldwide will experience more significant health equity, resilience, and collective flourishing. Investing in positive health will not just be a cost but a long-term strategy that will lead to healthier, more productive societies, reducing the burden on healthcare systems and fostering economic growth.

As more individuals embrace positive health, communities will transform. Rates of non-communicable diseases will plummet, and mental health will flourish. People of all ages will enjoy higher levels of wellbeing, resulting in a society that is not only healthier but also more connected and compassionate. Public health systems will see reduced burdens as preventative measures will become well established, leading to longer, healthier lives for all. These outcomes will be not just theoretical; they will be supported by numerous studies and real-world examples that demonstrate the effectiveness of positive health in improving health and wellbeing.

Positive health will become the cornerstone of public policy, with governments investing in community-based positive health initiatives that combine lifestyle medicine and positive psychology. These initiatives will foster environments that support healthy living and mental wellbeing, from parks and recreational facilities to community centres offering wellness programmes and mental health resources. By integrating positive health into public policy, governments will ensure the widespread adoption of these principles and practices, making them accessible to all.

Positive health will make the world a better place in this future vision. It will transcend boundaries and become a universal movement embraced by individuals, families, workplaces, schools, and governments. Integrating lifestyle medicine and positive psychology will create a synergistic effect, enhancing the quality of life and fostering a global culture of health and healthiness.

In this vision of the future, positive health will not just be a concept – it will be a way of life that will shape our society's collective outcomes. It will support us in times of uncertainty, and become a source of strength in times of adversity. Together, we will embark on a journey toward a world where health is not merely the absence of illness but the presence of vitality, joy, and fulfilment for all.

# INDEX

Note: Locators in *italic* indicate figures, in **bold** tables and in ***bold-italic*** boxes.

Printed in the United States
by Baker & Taylor Publisher Services